How You Can Live

Six Extra Years

How You Can Live

Six
Extra Years

*These simple proven steps
can add six or more years
to your life span—better,
happier years. Thousands
of people are doing it—
you can too!*

Lewis R. Walton, J.D.
Jo Ellen Walton, M.D.
John A. Scharffenberg, M.D.

Published by

Woodbridge Press Publishing Company
Santa Barbara, California 93111

Published by
Woodbridge Press Publishing Company
Post Office Box 6189
Santa Barbara, California 93111

Printed in the United States of America
Published simultaneously in Canada

Library of Congress Cataloging in Publication Data

Walton, Lewis R
  Six extra years.

  Bibliography: p.
  1. Diet.   2. Longevity—Nutritional aspects.   3. Seventh-Day
Adventists—Health and Hygiene.   I. Walton, Joe Ellen, joint author.
II. Scharffenberg, John A., joint author.   III. Title.
RA784.W34   613.2'6   80-28030
ISBN 0-912800-84-4

CONTENTS

Prologue

Last Chance for a Miracle

It is 5:40 A.M. and from my office window I can begin to see the Sierras, California's great eastern wall guarding the San Joaquin Valley. The mountains are bathed in the first promise of dawn, and I turn out my light to watch for a few moments, savoring the quiet that precedes the day. But it is an illusion and I know it. For me, the day has already begun.

I am a hospital attorney trying to keep my client alive.

And time is running out.

This particular day began several hours ago, with a problem that occurred at 1:30 A.M. Just as dawn colors the sky I wrap up the last loose ends. The hospital will survive to face another day, patched up like a ship that has no time to stop for real repairs. Now I stand by my desk, watching the sunrise, wondering if it is late or early. And finally I decide: it is late—very, very late. Unless we do something soon, America's health care system will collapse as a free institution.

In our intensive care unit this morning four patients are recovering from open heart surgery. The cost of their care will exceed $20,000 each. It represents a staggering burden, too expensive even for the richest nation on earth. Others, in our cancer wing, will spend long and expensive weeks in the hospital. Some of them will have only small odds of seeing the magical five-year survival that doctors call a "cure." The cost of cancer this year? Probably close to twenty-five *billion* dollars!

Few people realize how much we are paying because of poor health habits. Let me give you a vivid example. On my desk are two patient charts nearly identical in every respect—except for price and length of hospital stay. Both men were admitted on the same day. Each had the same abdominal surgery. But one patient was of normal size and the other was grossly overweight. The first man was

1

released after eight days in the hospital; his bill was $3,465. The overweight man stayed ten days. Because of poorer health he had a long, brutally expensive stay in intensive care. His bill? $6,054. That represents nearly 3,000 extra dollars for hospitalization alone—a terrible extra burden that was probably almost totally preventable.

These facts race through my mind and I silently ask myself a familiar question for which I have no answer: how much more pressure can the system stand? Year by year the cost of health care goes further off the end of the scale. Soon, unless some miracle occurs, the whole system will collapse. Medical care as we have come to expect it will simply be unavailable at any price.

But this morning I believe there may still be a solution. In the quiet hours of dawn, before the hospital wakes up and shatters my reverie, I recall some health study statistics that crossed my desk a few days ago. There is a group of people who use hospital services much less than do most Americans, according to the statistics. They have a dramatically lower risk of death from heart attack, stroke, and many cancers. In plain terms, they need less of the really expensive medical services that are bankrupting this country's health care system. They are Seventh-day Adventists. And this morning it occurs to me that Americans should take a second look at what they have been saying about health for over a hundred years.

This year alone Americans will spend $29 billion on heart and vascular disease. If everyone followed the Adventist health program we could cut that figure by more than half. Another $25 billion will go for cancers, for which Adventists enjoy a general risk reduction of 41 percent. We could probably save 750,000 lives a year and millions of needless hospitalizations if Americans would follow the basic, commonsense ideas Adventists have long advocated. And in the process they could expect an extra 6.2 years of life expectancy—good years, freer from disease, freer from the mental and physical debilities of old age. I think it is worth trying.

And so this morning I know what I have to do. In our hospital is a team of experts in public health, nutrition, and disease prevention. Concerned about the rising cost of health care, we have for four years been trying to cut those costs by telling people in Bakersfield how to live healthfully. Perhaps it is time to share that idea in a brotherly way—to tell the American people that there *is* a way out. It is called *prevention.* We *can* cut costs and ease human suffering.

5:45 A.M. I have been daydreaming for only five minutes. There is a sudden flash of light. Over the mountains an early summer sun rises into view and blasts our valley with a hue that promises heat. It is time to go to work.

Good morning to the city of Bakersfield.

> Lewis R. Walton
> General Counsel
> San Joaquin Community
>   Hospital Corporation

Chapter 1

The Evidence Is Overwhelming

In recent years research has uncovered exciting new evidence that disease, with all its human and economic costs, is surprisingly preventable.

Consider the following:

Studies show that an American man can reduce his heart attack risk by 85 percent.

Lung cancer risk can be reduced by 80 percent.

Women can reduce their risk of uterine cancer by 46 percent.

How do we know? Simply because a group of people in this country—the Seventh-day Adventists—have already done it.

For a number of years scientists have been interested in studying Adventist health. As a research population Adventists are useful, because they live within the American culture and geography, thereby eliminating many errors that can creep into comparisons of people from different nationalities. In many respects they are indistinguishable from other Americans, living and working in substantially the same environment as does everyone else. But there is a significant difference that intrigues researchers. For over 100 years Adventists have stressed the importance of health and diet, the necessity of moderation in the intake of foods high in sugar and saturated fat. While all Adventists do not follow the church's total diet and life-style program, enough do to offer some significant epidemiological comparisons. Given these factors, it was inevitable that they would be studied by health researchers.

The results are worth a second look. In nearly every major disease, Adventists rank well below the average in risk. Some of the differences are startling, such as the enormous reduction in heart attack risk for men who carefully follow their church's health ideas. Notice how the data in Figure 1 and Table 1 show Adventists' significant advantage for nearly every disease shown. Notice, too, in Figure 2 that the advantage seems to be directly related to how closely they adhere to the health program.

Figure 1

Death Rate of Seventh-day Adventists Due to Various Causes Compared with Those of the General Population

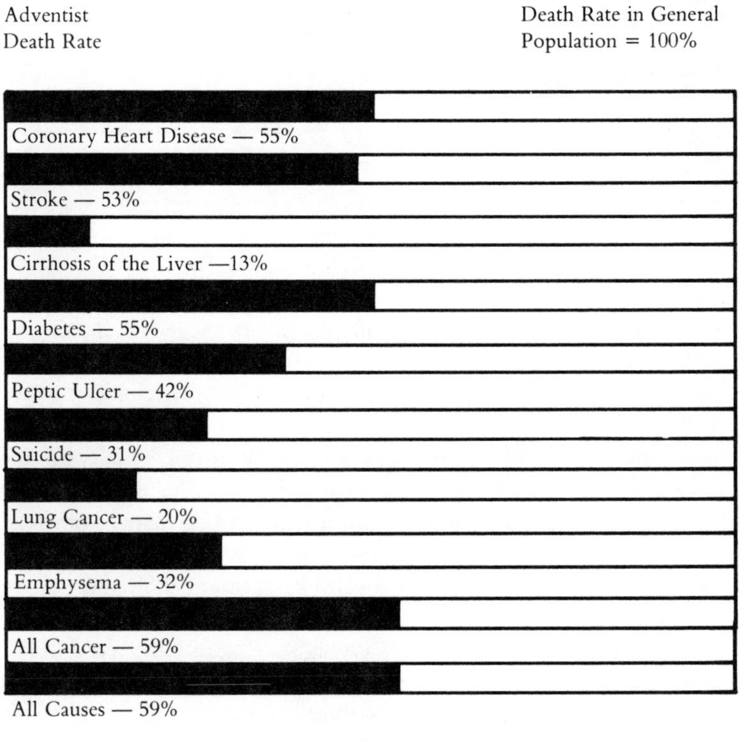

Adventist
Death Rate

Death Rate in General
Population = 100%

Coronary Heart Disease — 55%	
Stroke — 53%	
Cirrhosis of the Liver —13%	
Diabetes — 55%	
Peptic Ulcer — 42%	
Suicide — 31%	
Lung Cancer — 20%	
Emphysema — 32%	
All Cancer — 59%	

All Causes — 59%

Figure 2

Coronary Death Rate for Adventist Men with Various Dietary Habits Compared with the General Population

Adventist   Death Rate in General
Death Rate   Population = 100%

14% — Total vegetarian

39% — Vegetarian plus milk and eggs

56% — Meat included in diet

37% — Nonvegetarian

12% — Vegetarian

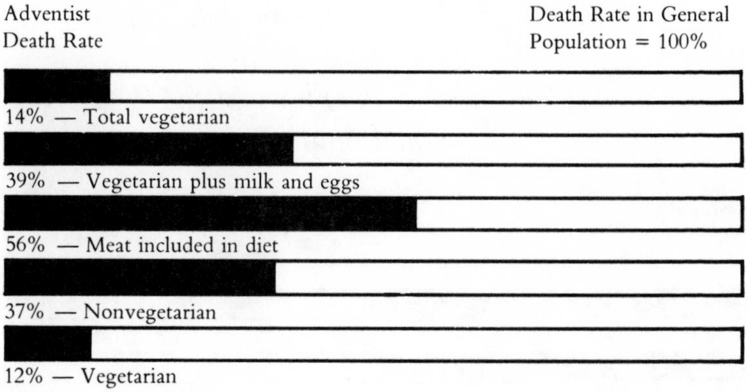

Perhaps the most intriguing statistic of all, especially for people in their retirement years, is life expectancy. From the data in Table 1 we can see that an Adventist man age 35–40 in California can expect to live over six years longer than his average California counterpart. And he will not only live longer, but probably live better during those six extra years; better general health softens many of the discomforts otherwise associated with old age. This increase in life expectancy is greater than all our public health efforts have accomplished for the general population in the past seventy years. One writer of retirement annuities recently complained that the surest way to lose money was to write an annuity for an Adventist senior citizen living in the country. A check of the obituary columns in Adventist denominational papers shows that the man is probably right: of the deaths listed, a large number comprise people born in the last twenty years of the nineteenth century.

Table 1

Life Expectancy

California Men	71 years
Adventist Men	77 years
California Women	77 years
Adventist Women	80 years

Since 1863 Adventists have been increasingly interested in proper health. One of their first great concerns was to limit intake of foods high in saturated fats. For the most part—then, as now—that means limiting one's intake of animal products, which are usually high in saturates and which, Adventists warned in 1870, could increase the risk of disease by "tenfold."[1] Hold that figure in your memory for the next few pages.

For many years the Adventist stand on diet aroused skepticism. The relationship between diet and disease was nearly incomprehensible to people in an age where even minor illnesses were routinely treated with strychnine, prussic acid, and occasional reversions to bloodletting. And, strange to say, the Adventist rationale continued to be largely ignored until quite recently when research results began coming in linking diet and heart disease.

In 1960 a team of researchers in Finland decided to study the relationship between saturated fat and heart disease. For six years men at one mental hospital were put on a diet where whole milk was replaced with skim milk, richened with the addition of polyunsaturated vegetable oil. Butter was changed to soft margarine. Otherwise, the diet remained the same. In another hospital a second group of patients continued to receive the usual high-saturated fat diet, including butter and whole milk. The results were significant. At the end of six years, death rates from coronary heart disease were cut in half among the men on the low-saturated fat diet.

Now the groups were switched. The men who had been getting whole milk and butter were given the vegetable oil substitutes, while the earlier "healthy" group went back to purely animal products. The result? After six more years, the new group on the low-saturated fat diet also enjoyed a reduction in heart attack death rate. Clearly there seemed to be a link between diet and heart disease.

Other experiments confirmed the Finnish results. Dr. Norman Jolliffe of New York completed a ten-year study he had begun back in 1957, with results nearly identical to those in Finland. In Los Angeles, researchers at the Veterans Administration Hospital split veterans living there into two groups, assigning them to two separate cafeterias. In one, polyunsaturates were used instead of saturated animal fats; in the other, the usual higher fat diet was continued. After eight years, coronary heart disease dropped by one-half in the group on a low-saturated fat diet.

Evidence continued to build. A study on heart disease rates in Norway showed that during the war, when animal fat consumption was low, the rate of circulatory disease also dropped. Another study compared the heart attack rate for men in Framingham, Massachusetts, with that for men living in Japan. The Japanese, on a traditionally low fat diet, enjoyed an advantage of eight to one.

But perhaps the most exciting statistics of all were published in 1979. Fifty thousand Seventh-day Adventists in California were surveyed by a team of university researchers. They completed comprehensive health questionnaires. Medical records were released and studied. Health statistics for Adventists were compared with those for average Californians. The results provided a surprise even for scientists who had expected to see a difference. Adventist men who were careful about following their dietary and life-style program had a heart attack mortality rate only *12 percent* that of the average California male. Their advantage was over eight to one. The evidence was overwhelming.

Now it is time to use the figure we asked you to remember. Recall that on page 7 we mentioned an early Adventist prediction of a "tenfold" increase in risk when certain animal products are used. In the case of heart disease, that figure is very nearly reached. And remember that this prediction was made in 1870, when sick babies were still being treated with a powerful emetic called "antimonial wine," given to induce violent vomiting because disease was thought to result from "too much vitality."

Thus far we have talked only of heart disease. What about other diseases that cost us lives and high hospital bills?

This year cancer will kill nearly 400,000 Americans. Another 700,000 will learn for the first time that they have the disease. Despite all the advances in medical science, we will still lose cancer patients this year at the rate of *one every eighty seconds.* Directly and indirectly, cancer will cost us $25 billion.

Table 2 shows Adventist cancer death rates compared with those in the general population. Notice that Adventists have a significantly lower risk of death from cancer. A number of scientists are beginning to wonder if this may be related to their low intake of meat.

Table 2

Cancer Death Rates—SDA's Compared With the General Population

Digestive Tract Cancer	65%
Leukemia	62%
Uterine Cancer	54%
Ovarian Cancer	61%
Lung Cancer	20%
Mouth, Throat, Larynx Cancer	5%
Bladder Cancer	28%

Perhaps no area of the Adventist health program has aroused more argument than their stand on the use of meat. While vegetarianism is not a religious dogma in the church (certain "clean" meats are allowed, and some Adventists eat them), a meat-free diet is still regarded as the ideal. In 1864, for example, the church published a caution that the use of meat could result in the onset of cancer growth. In 1909 church members were warned that "if meat eating was ever healthful, it is not safe now. *Cancers, tumors, and pulmonary diseases are largely caused by meat eating"* [italics supplied]. Such a statement was apt to provoke ridicule in 1909. But note the course of scientific discovery over the past seventy years. (In that day tuberculosis could well have been transmitted through diseased cattle, although that problem has now been eradicated in the United States.)

By interesting coincidence, just one year after Adventists received the above caution regarding transmittal of disease by meat, a researcher named Peyton Rous decided to see if cancer could be transmitted from one animal to another. He injected healthy chickens with fluids aspirated from hens known to have chicken sarcoma. The injected chickens came down with the same disease!

In 1936 Dr. Bittner carried this study one step further with his now famous demonstration that cancer can apparently be transmitted through the diet. He selected mice known to have breast tumors and allowed them to nurse young female mice who were free from the disease and whose parents had been free from it. Mammary tumors soon developed in the young nursing females. Apparently, cancer had been transmitted.

But many questions remained to be answered, and in the 1960s researchers decided to try a different approach. What about the transmissibility of cancer from one species to another? What about human cancer? To answer these questions they took leukemic tissue from human beings and injected it into small laboratory animals. The animals came down not with leukemia but with lung cancer, breast cancer, and several other forms of the disease—a frightening hint that some of these killers not only may pass from one species to another, but that they may also bear some undiscovered relationship between each other.

And then in 1974 the scientific community was jolted by a discovery made by a team of researchers who had decided to try a variation of Dr. Bittner's 1936 study. They took six chimpanzees, whose physiology is similar to humans, and from birth onward, fed them formulas using milk from known leukemic cows. *Within one year, two of the test animals had died from leukemia.*

Conclusive evidence of the danger of cancer from diet? Not totally. But it comes close enough to provoke this ominous remark in the American Cancer Society's *Journal:* "Comment to stimulate a sense of urgency appears superfluous." In other words, watch out.

Now to put things into perspective, let us quote from one more Adventist warning on the use of meat, this one given back in 1905: "People are continually eating flesh that is filled with tuberculous and cancerous germs. Tuberculosis, cancer, and other fatal diseases are thus communicated."[3] A startling statement, to be sure, made 5 years before Peyton Rous introduced the first glimmer of the cancer virus theory, 31 years before Bittner, 69 years before the study that proved that leukemia may be transmissible through an agent as seemingly innocent as milk. (Adventists have long urged that if milk is used, it should be well cooked.) It is difficult to imagine people being further ahead of their time.

Heart disease, cancer, strokes—even peptic ulcers. The results are there, and the percentages are too great to explain away as statistical error. Whatever Adventists are doing, it must be right; the statistics are too persuasive to allow much room for argument.

The evidence is in, and the evidence is overwhelming.

And now to the big question: How do they do it?

Chapter 2

Diet: What, When, and How

Most Americans do not realize how much of their present dietary heritage is the product of Adventist innovation. Peanut butter. Meat substitutes such as imitation bacon and sausage. Corn flakes. (Yes, corn flakes were invented by an Adventist named Kellogg.) The entire multibillion-dollar breakfast cereal industry. Even soy milk, which has saved the lives of thousands of infants allergic to cow's milk.

All of these were the product of Adventists, caught in a world that does not fit their strict dietary standards, and hence utilizing their own brand of Yankee ingenuity to fill the gaps.

But the Adventist concept of diet goes far beyond the topic of what to eat. It also tells how to eat, and when—and even where. It describes combinations of foods that are best avoided. It advises on the most helpful ways to cook. It even describes an intricate link between the digestive system and the brain, reaching the conclusion that people's mental acuity, efficiency, and even happiness hinge to a remarkable degree on how they follow the rules of diet. It is a comprehensive approach, and we begin by looking at their answer to one of America's greatest public health problems today, the misuse of sugar.

SUGAR

Each year every man, woman and child in America consumes, per capita, over 125 pounds of refined sugar. In simple terms, that means that many Americans are actually eating their weight in sugar each year. The results show—in epidemic levels of tooth decay, in overweight and diabetes, and in many other diseases that scientists are beginning to link to high sugar consumption. We will talk shortly about the problems sugar causes. But first let's talk about how to handle the sugar problem itself.

The Adventist approach to sugar is quite simple and can be condensed into two basic rules: carefully limit the use of sugar, and especially avoid combining it with milk or eggs. The reasons for these rules are physiologically interesting, and we'll discuss them one at a time.

Limit the use of sugar. As early as 1870, Adventists were warned, in interesting graphic language that: "sugar clogs the system. It hinders the working of the living machine."[1]

Is there any scientific evidence that their belief may be right? Dental researchers have done a study that sheds light on this. Inside the tooth are spaces in which fluids normally circulate: the health of the tooth in part depends on this free circulation. Using sophisticated color photographic techniques, researchers have been able to observe the fluid movement in the teeth of laboratory animals before and after they consumed large quantities of sugar. The result? After the use of sugar, the fluid movement in the teeth is dramatically lessened. Researchers now feel that this may be representative of what sugar does in other parts of the body. There probably is no better one-syllable way to say it than that sugar "clogs" the system.

For these reasons, Adventists advise cutting the use of sugar to a bare minimum. Some sugar is admittedly useful in canning and preserving food, and for making certain dishes appetizing. Nor do they condemn sugar in an occasional dessert, taken in moderation. But as a general rule the serious Adventist health reformer will try to remove as much sugar as possible from the diet.

Table 3

Some Hidden Sources of Sugar★

Food	Size Portion	Teaspoons
Cola drinks	1 (6-ounce bottle)	3½
Ginger ale	1 (6-ounce bottle)	5
Orange-ade	1 (8-ounce glass)	5
Soda pop	1 (8-ounce glass)	5
Angel food cake	1 piece (4 ounces)	7

Food	Size Portion	Teaspoons
Banana cake	1 piece (2 ounces)	2
Chocolate cake, plain	1 piece (4 ounces)	6
Chocolate cake, iced	1 piece (4 ounces)	10
Coffee cake	1 piece (4 ounces)	4½
Cup cake, iced	1	6
Fruit or pound cake	1 piece (4 ounces)	5
Jelly-roll	1 piece (2 ounces)	2½
Sponge cake	1 piece (1 ounce)	2
Strawberry shortcake	1 serving	4
Brownies, unfrosted	1 (¾ ounce)	3
Chocolate cookies	1	1½
Fig newtons	1	5
Ginger snaps	1	3
Macaroons	1	6
Nut cookies	1	1½
Oatmeal cookies	1	2
Chocolate eclair	1	7
Cream puff	1	2
Doughnut, plain	1	3
Doughnut, glazed	1	6
Chocolate milk bar	1 (1½ ounces)	2½
Chewing gum	1 stick	½
Chocolate cream	1 piece	2
Butterscotch chew	1 piece	1
Fudge	1 ounce square	4½
Gum drop	1	2
Hard candy	1 ounce (5 pieces)	5
Peanut brittle	1	3½
Canned apricots	4 halves & 1 tablespoon syrup	3½
Canned fruit juices, sweetened	½ cup	2
Canned peaches	2 halves & 1 tablespoon syrup	3½
Stewed fruits	½ cup	2
Ice cream	¼ pint (3½ ounces)	3½
Ice cream bar	1	1–7
Ice cream cone	1	3½
Ice cream sundae	1	7
Malted milk shake	1 (10-ounce glass)	5
Apple butter	1 tablespoon	1
Jelly or marmalade	1 tablespoon	4–6
Strawberry jam	1 tablespoon	4
Apple cobbler	½ cup	3

Custard	½ cup	2
French pastry	1 (4-ounce piece)	5
Jello	½ cup	4½
Apple pie	1 slice, average	7
Butterscotch pie	1 slice	4
Cherry or berry pie	1 slice	10
Cream pie	1 slice	4
Lemon pie	1 slice	7
Mince meat pie	1 slice	4
Pumpkin pie	1 slice	5
Rhubarb pie	1 slice	4
Chocolate or plum pudding	½ cup	4
Rice pudding	½ cup	5
Tapioca pudding or brown betty	½ cup	3
Berry tart	1	10
Sherbet	½ cup	9
Chocolate icing	1 ounce	5
Chocolate sauce	1 tablespoon	3½
Corn or Karo syrup	1 tablespoon	3
Granulated sugar or honey	1 tablespoon	3
Maple syrup	1 tablespoon	5
Molasses	1 tablespoon	3½

*From American Foundation for Medical-Dental Science, Los Angeles, California.

How?

First, read labels. Sugar comes to us in modern food in every imaginable form. It comes openly, in the doughnuts we have at coffee breaks. It comes partially hidden, in the form of cola drinks, most of which contain at least five teaspoons of it. It also arrives, cleverly disguised, in such innocent substances as dry breakfast cereals, some of which contain up to 68 percent refined sugar. (That's right: 68 percent. Check the label on most dry breakfast cereals and you will find sugar as the second ingredient, right behind grain. Check some of them, and you will find sugar listed *first*.) Reading and understanding food labels is one of the first habits a careful food shopper should develop, and Adventists have developed it to a refined art.

Substitute naturally sweet foods such as fruit. Fruit offers many advantages as a food. It is naturally tasty and hence does not need

Figure 3

Annual Per Capita
Sugar Consumption in the United States

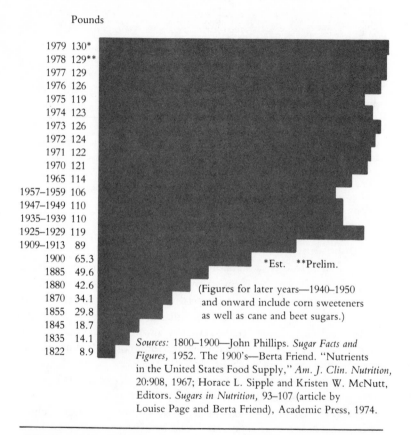

Pounds

1979	130*
1978	129**
1977	129
1976	126
1975	119
1974	123
1973	126
1972	124
1971	122
1970	121
1965	114
1957–1959	106
1947–1949	110
1935–1939	110
1925–1929	119
1909–1913	89
1900	65.3
1885	49.6
1880	42.6
1870	34.1
1855	29.8
1845	18.7
1835	14.1
1822	8.9

*Est.   **Prelim.

(Figures for later years—1940–1950
and onward include corn sweeteners
as well as cane and beet sugars.)

Sources: 1800–1900—John Phillips. *Sugar Facts and Figures,* 1952. The 1900's—Berta Friend. "Nutrients in the United States Food Supply," *Am. J. Clin. Nutrition,* 20:908, 1967; Horace L. Sipple and Kristen W. McNutt, Editors. *Sugars in Nutrition,* 93–107 (article by Louise Page and Berta Friend), Academic Press, 1974.

additives such as sugar, salt, and other substances that are so often overused in food. It also has very little fat content, no cholesterol, and is low in sodium, so it can be enjoyed by most people who have heart disease or high blood pressure problems. And it has considerably fewer calories per serving than do prepared sweets.

For those persons who find it hard to give up more traditional sweets such as pastries, Adventists have come up with recipes for sugarless cookies, bear claws, even pies, using only the sweetening found in natural fruits. Some of these are given in the Appendix.

Especially avoid combining sugar, milk, and eggs. Adventists believe that the effects of sugar are greatly worsened when combined with milk, cream, or eggs. Overindulgence in this combination can produce indigestion in many people (a child's stomachache after a birthday party being a conspicuous example). But even more importantly, there may be a link between this combination of foods and more serious diseases.

To understand this, one has to understand how sugar affects the body's mechanism for fighting disease. In the bloodstream there are special fighter cells (called white cells) whose major function is to surround and immobilize bacteria and other agents of disease, destroying them before a person becomes ill. Most of the time they function with awesome ability. Each day we are probably exposed to scores of diseases; usually we never even realize that this has happened, because the white blood cells have attacked the intruders before they can do real harm. But sugar has a strange, paralyzing effect on white blood cells. They become sluggish, inept, able to deal with only a fraction of the bacteria they normally handle.

When rats are given sugar equivalent to a human eating as little as six teaspoons—slightly more than one cola drink—their disease-fighting ability is reduced by 25 percent. Twelve teaspoons knock out 60 percent. Twenty-four teaspoons of sugar bring their germ-fighting abilities almost to total collapse, reducing them by 92 percent. In humans that is the same vulnerability found in an uncontrolled diabetic. Physicians who treat diabetics have a healthy respect for their susceptibility to infectious disease. They are often at the mercy of common infections. They have four to five times greater risk of contracting tuberculosis. And it appears possible for any healthy individual to temporarily lower his or her resistance to that level, simply by eating twenty-four teaspoons of refined sugar at a sitting. Impossible to do? Hardly. The average banana split has twenty-five!

Now let's return to an early Adventist warning about milk and sugar, given back in 1870: "Large quantities of milk and sugar eaten together are injurious. They impart impurities to the system."[2] Milk is an ideal culture medium for bacteria. Even pasteurization, as helpful as it is, falls far short of sterilization. And as milk is added during food preparation there are many opportunities for bacteria to enter even if they were not originally present. Now combine the presence of virile, growing bacteria cultures with sugar, which depresses the body's bacteria fighting ability, and you have an instant answer to the question of why sore throats and other illnesses so often seem to follow a large ice cream sundae or a second piece of cake.

You also have a scientific basis for the concern that Adventists have expressed since 1870.

Some scientists now feel that milk and sugar combinations may also increase one's risk of diabetes. Milk has been shown to stimulate the production of certain hormones within the body. When these hormones are given to laboratory animals together with carbohydrates such as sugar, the ultimate result is diabetes.

Sugar alone may also be associated with diabetes. A number of studies have been done that seem to suggest that link. For example, Yemenite Jewish immigrants to Israel had a low incidence of diabetes until they had consumed a Westernized diet high in sugar for several years.[3]

There are other reasons for Adventists' concern over combining milk, eggs, and sugar. The butterfat in milk and cream contains a high proportion of saturated animal fat. Scientists now know that saturated fat in the diet causes blood cholesterol levels to go up. Cholesterol is a thick, waxy substance and perhaps we can think of it behaving in the bloodstream something like wet cement. It settles onto the vulnerable lining of the arteries, slowly building up and hardening until the artery feels, through a surgeon's glove, like a tiny tube of stone. (The term *"hardened arteries"* is really quite descriptive.) Thus, when butterfat is taken into the body, levels of cholesterol in the bloodstream usually tend to rise. Now enters the second villain, sugar. Some studies show that excess sugar tends to raise blood levels of fats known as triglycerides. Many scientists believe that these fats actually cause cholesterol to deposit in the arteries more rapidly. One problem thus compounds another.

It is time to introduce the third villain, animal cholesterol. We have already seen that saturated fat causes elevated blood cholesterol. When you take additional cholesterol from some animal source, such as eggs, you have a third problem piled atop an already bad situation. Egg yolk contains so much cholesterol, that many physicians now urge their patients to eat no more than two eggs per week, and heart patients to eat no egg yolks at all. The combination of milk, sugar, and eggs produces a veritable witch's brew of problems: cholesterol levels rise, additional animal cholesterol is added, and the whole sticky mess is sent into the arterial lining by the addition of sugar. Blood cholesterol is elevated more rapidly by a combination of cholesterol, saturated fat, and sugar than by any one of them alone. Probably one could not summarize the situation better than by simply saying that "sugar clogs the system."

Finally, what about other serious diseases such as cancer? Recall that in chapter 1 we mentioned a 1974 study in which healthy chimpanzees, fed milk from leukemic cows, died within a year from leukemia. Admittedly, most milk is pasteurized. But is pasteurization sufficient to kill the powerful viruses that may be associated with leukemia? We don't know. And what about eggs? It is common knowledge among researchers that from 5 to 10 percent of the eggs produced in the American poultry industry carry leukosis, a form of cancer. Ordinary cooking is thought to destroy the virus, but we have learned through hard experience that viruses can be remarkably unpredictable. In the 1950s for example, a number of children came down with polio after being injected with what was thought to be a perfectly harmless, killed vaccine.

Does the Adventist position on sugar square with current scientific thinking? Yes, and rather decidedly so. In 1977 the Senate Select Committee on Nutrition and Human Needs published a report expressing concern that we are "displacing complex carbohydrates, which are high in micronutrients, with sugar, which is essentially an energy source offering little other nutritional value."[4] The report warned that we are thus depriving ourselves of essential micronutrients while taking in sugar calories which "may actually increase the body's need for certain vitamins."[5] For example, sugar may increase the need for thiamin, which is needed to metabolize it, together with trace elements such as chromium. In simple terms, the nutritional effect is a downward spiral. Scientists have come up with a very descriptive term to characterize the process: empty calories.

How should we handle the sugar problem? The Senate Select Committee offers suggestions surprisingly similar to those the Adventists have urged since the turn of the century.

Reduce soft drink consumption.

Reduce consumption of high sugar bakery goods.

Shop wisely. Notice the data in Table 3 showing the hidden sources of sugar in U.S. foods.

Sugar has become such an important part of food marketing that it is difficult to find even a breakfast cereal that is low in sugar. The problem has reached a point where some cereals have more sugars than grain. Read the labels!

Adventist cautions about sugar, given in 1870, seem to be in the very mainstream of current scientific thought.

FIBER

One of the most exciting new developments in nutrition research is the discovery that fiber may greatly lessen the risk of many serious diseases. Heart disease, colon cancer, and even diverticulitis may all be diseases whose risk can be appreciably lowered simply by getting adequate fiber in the diet.

What do we know about fiber today?

It can speed the digestive transit time by over 250 percent. For millions of Americans who are dependent on laxatives and expensive food supplements, that fact alone ought to recommend it.

It may be an important way to lessen one's risk of heart disease. Many researchers now feel that fiber acts as a vehicle to carry off excess bile acids and cholesterol, which would otherwise be reabsorbed and trigger a cholesterol build-up. If that is so, then the Adventist preoccupation with whole grains, long out of fashion in an era of white bread and bleached pastry flour, will prove to be in the very mainstream of cardiovascular research.

It may also lessen one's risk of digestive tract cancer. Some bile acids, when present in excess, have been shown to cause digestive tract cancer in laboratory animals. With our modern high-fat, high-meat diet, the liver is stimulated to produce those acids in greater than normal quantities. Still other substances used as meat preservatives also react within the bowel to form carcinogens. The result is a potent combination of chemicals which, on the typical low-fiber diet, has nearly three full days in which to act on the lining of the digestive tract—over twice as long as in a person who eats a high-fiber diet. It should come as no surprise that colon cancer is our number two cancer killer in America today. It is surpassed only by cancer of the lung.

How do Adventists solve the dietary fiber problem? With one simple rule:

Include in the diet adequate quantities of fruits, vegetables, and whole grains, prepared simply and as nearly in the natural state as possible.

This rule does not imply a diet of raw or unappetizing food. What it does suggest is fresh food, as far as possible, and it urges the use of food before the fiber, vitamins, and vital trace elements have been milled out of it by a food processor. The idea has much to commend it. It supplies the best source of vitamins and minerals. It also gives the very best source of natural fiber, and may explain why Adventists enjoy a reduction of 35 percent in the risk of death from digestive tract cancer. (Believe it or not, Americans are now paying premium prices for expensive "high-fiber" foods in which the fiber content is bolstered with wood cellulose. There is probably nothing dangerous about eating wood by-products, but one would be tempted to ask why you are willing to pay extra for sawdust when you could accomplish just as much with vegetables and whole grains.)

Adventist advice on fiber and on the use of unrefined foods is beginning to be echoed by more and more responsible scientists. Dr. Denis Burkitt, one of the first advocates of the high-fiber diet, suggests that increased fiber consumption will markedly reduce the incidence of bowel cancer and other intestinal diseases. He urges that fiber be taken in unrefined foods rather than as an additive to refined products such as white bread.

Others have reported wide-ranging benefits from dietary fiber. Dr. Kenneth Heaton, of Britain's University of Bristol, reported that when he and his wife increased their fiber intake they noted a corresponding steady, effortless weight loss—accomplished without any conscious effort to count calories or restrict food intake. Studies done in Europe have produced similar results. Still other benefits from fiber reported by researchers are reduction of gall bladder disease, reduction of insulin requirements in diabetics, and reduction of distress in irritable bowel patients. Much more work needs to be done before conclusions can be drawn in some of these cases, but a general conclusion can safely be stated: for a variety of reasons, fiber in the diet is important.[6]

Adventist concern over getting food "as nearly in the natural state as possible" is not just a fetish. Consider the following illustrations. To get fiber equal to that of one fresh orange, one must drink over one quart of orange juice. To get the same amount of fiber found in one apple, it is necessary to drink half a gallon of apple juice. (The fiber present in whole apples tends to slow sugar absorption so that one does not get the reactive hypoglycemic response that might occur when using more refined products such as applesauce or apple juice.) To get the fiber obtainable in five slices of whole wheat bread, one would have to consume forty slices of white bread—two full loaves! Adventists see nothing wrong with fruit juices. Indeed, juices—prepared in a variety of interesting combinations—are the alternative they offer youngsters for soft drinks. Nor do they see anything wrong with an occasional switch to white bakery goods for the sake of variety. But their point is clear: anytime we process food, however innocuous that may seem to be, we run the risk of altering it and of removing much that is necessary: vitamins, minerals, and fiber, now acknowledged by scientists to be of great importance in preventing disease.

Table 4

Percentage of Calories from Foods with Little Fiber

Meat	20%
Refined cereals	18
Visible fats	18
Sugar	17
Milk	12
Alcohol	2
Eggs	2

SATURATED FAT

When Seventh-day Adventists first became concerned with what they called "health reform," the term *saturated fat* was not yet in use. If you could go back to 1863 and mention the term to an Adventist of that era, he—like other Americans of the 1860s—would respond with a blank stare. But interestingly, one of the significant results of early Adventist dietary reform was a reduction of saturated fat in the diet.

We are discovering that saturated fat plays a role in several serious diseases. It is clearly linked to heart and vascular disease. It is also becoming linked with cancer of the breast and colon. To the surprise of many researchers, it is emerging as an extremely broad-spectrum health hazard, implicated in illnesses we never guessed had anything to do with fat intake.

Excess dietary fat poses many problems. Fat is our most concentrated source of food energy—nearly twice as high in calories per gram as protein and carbohydrates. Consequently, for those who are not physically active it can be nearly impossible to control weight while eating the typical American diet with 40 percent of one's calories in the form of fat. Overweight, in turn, leads to a whole spectrum of risks: cardiovascular disease, high blood pressure, atherosclerosis, hernia, gallbladder disease, diabetes, liver diseases, and greatly increased risk of complications after surgery.

The link between dietary fat and cancer is also coming into focus. In 1976 Dr. Gio Gori, deputy director of the National Cancer Institute, said that there is a "strong correlation between dietary fat intake and incidence of breast cancer and colon cancer. . . . Colon cancer has also been shown to correlate highly with the consumption of meat, even though it is not clear whether the meat itself or its fat content is the real correlating factor."[7]

Scientists have become so alarmed about the relationship between saturated fat and disease that they now are beginning to urge a reduction of saturated fat to no more than 10 percent of one's daily calories. That is an astonishingly low figure. On the typical American diet it is highly difficult to achieve. And yet, Adventists have designated a program that can reach this goal—and which may help to account for their remarkably low incidence of heart attack and other fat-related diseases.

How do Seventh-day Adventists solve the saturated fat problem? Here are the rules they follow:

Substitute vegetable oils and margarines for high-fat dairy products. As early as 1873 Adventists were warned that butter should be phased out of the diet, and that its use was particularly harmful in children. (Autopsies done on American casualties in recent wars show that of our 22-year-olds, over one in ten *already* had 50 percent blockage of their coronary arteries, probably due to a high-animal fat diet.) Long ago Adventists were advised to use vegetable substitutes such as olive oil instead of butter. Today the food industry has caught up with those early concerns, and we have a wealth of polyunsaturated foods to choose from. Here are some practical suggestions Adventists frequently follow:

If milk is used, buy nonfat milk and richen it, if necessary, with a polyunsaturated nondairy creamer. But be careful. Some dairy substitutes are worse than the real thing. Coconut oil, one of the most saturated of all vegetable fats, is further saturated by artificial hydrogenation. The result is a product more saturated than cream. (The reason? Long shelf life.) Read the labels carefully, and notice the ratio between saturates and polyunsaturates in the product. When coconut oil or palm oil is high on the list of ingredients, beware!

Try making your own corn oil mayonnaise and substituting it for mayonnaise and sour cream. Actually, the product is not mayonnaise at all, since it contains no eggs, but is a tasty sauce that goes well on everything from tomato sandwiches to baked potatoes; the recipe is in the Appendix. Be especially cautious about commercial sour cream substitutes, which often contain heavily hydrogenated coconut oil and are thus more saturated than sour cream itself.

Use 100 percent corn oil margarine instead of butter—and use less of it.

When cooking, use only unsaturated vegetable oils, and use them sparingly. A little soy lecithin can replace some of the oil in your baking, thus reducing the amount of fat you get. Another suggestion: use a glass or plastic cooking oil dispenser that will help you to use drops instead of spoonfuls, and (if you must fry) you'll have lessened the fat that is used.

Try replacing eggs with tofu, an oriental product made from soy beans and exceptionally high in protein. It can be scrambled just like eggs, and when properly seasoned tastes so much like them that many people cannot tell the difference. The bonus for you? No cholesterol and very, very little saturated fat. The recipe is in the Appendix.

Avoid chips and other convenience foods, which, for the sake of shelf life, may be deep fried in highly saturated vegetable oil or lard. (Saturated oils oxidize—become rancid—more slowly and are therefore favored by many food processors because products "keep" on the shelf longer.) Many people in our hospital weight control classes find that the difference between weight loss and frustration can often be found in eliminating foods such as chips.

Eliminate lard and grease. The use of lard and pork products is one area where Adventists are dogmatic: they uniformly condemn them. Interestingly, this fits the pattern of Adventist concern over fat; pork products contain large amounts of saturated fat. A serious Adventist health reformer also will favor boiled or baked potatoes, for example, over french fries. Frying is generally avoided where some other

Table 5

Comparison of Nutrients in Tofu vs. Eggs (both scrambled)

	Per 100 calories		Per 100 grams	
	Scrambled Tofu	Scrambled Eggs	Scrambled Tofu	Scrambled Eggs
	1 cake 2¾" x 2½" x 1"= 85 calories	1 egg=77 calories	1 cake=1 lb. (454 gms) 100 gms=¼ cake	1 egg=54 gms 100 gms= almost 2 eggs
Water content (%)	84.8	72.1	84.8	72.1
Protein, gms	10.8	6.5	7.8	11.2
Fat, gms	5.8	7.5	4.2	12.9
Saturated fat, gms	0.9	2.4	0.6	4.1
P/S ratio	2.0	0.5	2.0	0.5
Cholesterol, mg	0	350.0	0	500.0
Calcium, mg	178.0	46.0	128.0	80.0
Iron, mg	2.6	1.0	1.9	1.7
Sodium, mg	10.0	149.0	7.0	257.0
Thiamine, mg	0.08	0.05	0.06	0.08
Riboflavin, mg	0.04	0.16	0.03	0.28
Vitamin A, I.U.	0	624.0	0	1080.0

form of cooking can be used, simply because grease is so prevalent in fried foods. (If you like hash browns, try this hint: cook them in your Teflon waffle iron without oil.)

Replace eggs with other protein sources. A large egg contains 250 milligrams of cholesterol together with quite a bit of saturated fat. Adventists have long taught that the safest practice is to learn to cook without eggs. They can be replaced with high-quality vegetable proteins that have no cholesterol such as tofu (see Table 5).

Cholesterol is only one reason why careful Adventists prefer not to use eggs. Recall that some of the commercial poultry in the United States is infected with a form of poultry cancer. The virus is present in the eggs. Ordinary cooking is thought to destroy the virus, and

Table 6

Saturated Fatty Acids in Selected Foods

Food	Saturated fatty acids	
	% of fat	Grams
Meat, poultry, fish		
Beef, cooked, 3 ounces	50	8
Hamburger	47	8
Round	46	6
Steak, sirloin	48	13
Roast, rib	47	16
Veal	54	6
Lamb chop, with bone, 4.8 ounces	55	18
Pork chop, with bone, 3.5 ounces	38	8
Ham, 3 ounces	39	7
Chicken, fryer, 3 ounces	32	2–3
Hen, 3 ounces	34	7
Fish sticks, 3.2 ounces	25	2
Salmon, 3 ounces	20	1
Dairy products and eggs		
Milk, whole, 1 cup	56	5
2%, 1 cup	56	3
Canned, evaporated, 1 tablespoon	56	0.7
Cheese, cheddar, 1 ounce	56	5
Cottage, creamed, 1/4 cup	56	1.5
Cream, 1 ounce	56	5

Food	% of fat	Grams
Cream, half & half, 1 tablespoon	56	1
Whipping, heavy, 1 tablespoon	56	3
Ice cream, 1/2 cup	56	4
Egg, large	33	2
Nuts and seeds		
Nuts, almonds, 1 ounce (not roasted)	8	1
Cashews, 1 ounce (roasted)	17	2
Peanuts, 1 ounce (roasted)	22	3
Coconut, 1 ounce	85	9
Peanut butter, 1 tablespoon	25	2
Walnuts, 1 ounce	5	1
Sunflower seeds, 1 ounce	13	2
Fats and oils		
Butter, 1 tablespoon	56	6.5
Lard, 1 tablespoon	38	5
Margarine, soft, 1 tablespoon	18	2
Oils, corn, 1 tablespoon	10	1.4
Olive, 1 tablespoon	11	1.5
Soybean, 1 tablespoon	15	2
Peanut, 1 tablespoon	18	2.5
Cottonseed, 1 tablespoon	25	3.5
Mayonnaise, 1 tablespoon	18	2
Salad dressings, 1 tablespoon	13	1
Desserts and sweets		
Cake, 1 piece	33	1–3
Candy, 1 ounce	27	3
Chocolate covered peanuts	25	3
Fudge, plain	50	2
Cookies, 1 average	33	1
Danish pastry, 4¼ inches in diameter	33	5
Ice cream, 1/2 cup	56	4
Pudding, average, 1 cup	50	5
Miscellaneous		
Avocado, 1/2 medium	19	3.5
Macaroni and cheese, 1 cup	45	10
Pizza with cheese, 2½ ounces	33	2
Pancake	50	1
Waffle, 7 inch diameter	29	2
Soup, cream, 1 cup	30	3–4
Soybeans, cooked, 1/2 cup	20	1

may. But are we absolutely sure? Many Adventists reason that there is no point in testing the hypothesis so long as high-quality substitutes are so readily available.

Adventists are not the only ones who are concerned about the use of eggs. One famed nutritionist has said that "it is time we relegated eggs back to the biological purpose for which they were designed." Many doctors recommend no more than two eggs per week. The Senate Select Committee on Nutrition and Human Needs has urged Americans to "decrease consumption of butterfat, eggs, and other high cholesterol sources."[8]

Substitute high-quality, low-fat entrees for meat. We will not talk in detail now about meat and meat substitutes, since that important topic is coming up next as a separate item. But it is important to remember that meat is one of the greatest sources of hidden fat in the diet. For many people it is probably the single greatest source of saturated fat. Take a look at Table 8, which shows the fat content of foods, starting with those highest in saturated fat. Surprised at the foods at the top of the list? So were many researchers. But the figures help to explain why Americans suffer from so many fat-related illnesses. By replacing meat with low-fat foods, Adventists have been able to beat those statistics by up to 800 percent. How they do it, and what foods they use as high-protein entrees, will be our next topic.

Table 7

Ratio of Polyunsaturates to Saturates in Meat★

1. Fish	2.0–3.0
2. Turkey	0.83
3. Chicken	0.81
4. Bacon	0.47
5. Luncheon meats	0.39
6. Deer	0.13
7. Lamb	0.07
8. Goat	0.07
9. Beef	0.06

★The higher figures show more polyunsaturates are present.

Table 8

Sources of Fat in the U.S. Diet

Food group	% of total fat
Meat (including poultry and fish)	34.2
Cooking and salad oils	14.5
Shortening	13.2
Dairy products (excluding butter)	12.9
Margarine	7.2
Legumes and cocoa	5.0
Butter	3.1
Eggs	3.0
Lard (direct use)	2.7
Other edible fats and oils	1.9
Grain products	1.4
Fruits and vegetables	0.9
	100.0

MEAT

Today we are witnessing one of the most fascinating revolutions ever seen in the nutritional world. Many people are beginning to suggest that there may be problems with meat, a food we have always assumed should be part of every meal.

Meat—staple food of the western frontier. Fortunes were made on it (and still are). We have become so accustomed to it that we are shocked when scientists suggest that it is implicated in some of our most serious diseases. But in 1970, the prestigious Inter-Society Commission for Heart Disease Resources, a group composed of twenty-nine health agencies, including the American Medical Association, made a startling suggestion. They said that Americans should avoid egg yolks, bacon, lard, and suet. They suggested that we eat more grains, fruits, vegetables and legumes. And they concluded, "It is necessary to encourage further developments of high quality vegetable protein products."[9] What is so significant about that statement? It describes exactly the program Adventists have been urging since 1863.

More recently, in February 1977, the Senate Select Committee on Nutrition and Human Needs published a report entitled *Dietary*

Goals for the United States. Predictably, it met stormy opposition from the powerful meat- and food-processing industries because it dared to face some sensitive issues. Our high-meat, high-sugar diet, the committee warned, "is everywhere associated with a similar disease pattern—high rates of coronary heart disease, certain forms of cancer, diabetes, and obesity."[10] Sound familiar? In chapter 1 we quoted a surprisingly similar Adventist statement from 1909: "If meat eating was ever healthful, it is not safe now. Cancers, tumors, and pulmonary diseases are largely caused by meat eating."[11]

Let's explore some of the problems with meat, as Adventists see them, and then we'll show how they maintain sound nutrition without it.

Heart disease. We quote from an Adventist book on health compiled in 1897: "Both the blood and the fat of animals is consumed as a luxury. But . . . these should not be eaten. Why?—Because their use would make a diseased current of blood in the human system."[12]

What do we know about the physiological effects of meat in the diet? First, as we have already seen, it contains large quantities of saturated fat. When this is taken into the system it elevates blood cholesterol, a disastrous surplus that circulates in the bloodstream and settles into the lining of the arteries. Meat aggravates this problem in a couple of other ways. First, it contains cholesterol of its own, thus adding to the body's surplus. Secondly, a diet high in meat is usually low in fiber. (As fibrous as it may seem to be, meat contains none of the lignin, pectin, cellulose, or hemicellulose that are found only in plants and are necessary for healthy bowel function.) Fiber in the bowel is now thought to act as a vehicle that removes excess bile acids from the body. If these acids are not removed, they are recycled and trigger still higher blood cholesterol levels. Remember that the final destination for much of the human body's excess cholesterol is the bloodstream, where it burdens the vulnerable arteries with sometimes fatal results.

Now reflect on the historical Adventist statement that the use of meat, with its blood and fat, causes a "diseased current of blood in the human system." That is a pretty graphic description of a condition that could precede coronary heart disease.

The effects of meat eating on heart disease death rates can be seen quite vividly among Adventists themselves. Remember that not all

Adventists follow their church's health program. Some do eat meat, and their heart attack incidence runs well above that of those who do not. Table 9 shows heart attack mortality among three groups of Adventist men: those who use no animal products, those who use milk and eggs, and those who eat meat. As one departs from the health program, there is almost a straight-line increase in risk.

Table 9

Seventh-day Adventist Coronary Death Rates

Total vegetarian	14% of the usual death rate
Vegetarian & milk, eggs	39% of the usual death rate
Nonvegetarian	56% of the usual death rate

Cancer. Consider the following statement from the book *Counsels on Diet and Foods,* a 500-page Adventist book devoted entirely to nutrition: "People are continually eating flesh that is filled with cancerous germs." The result? "Cancer and other fatal diseases are thus communicated."[13]

What do we know about meat and cancer today? Some forms of cancer are known to bear a high relationship to one's intake of meat. Other cancers are related to fat, much of which is obtained through a high-meat diet. Both colon cancer and breast cancer have been shown to relate to one's intake of beef, pork, and other meats.

The problem with colon cancer is thought to stem from chemical carcinogens created in the colon as a result of a high-meat diet. It appears that meat may cause the liver to produce excess bile acids. Meat also contains cholesterol. It is thought that both cholesterol and bile acids may be converted to powerful cancer-causing substances. Meat's lack of fiber aggravates the problem, because in the absence of fiber the food moves sluggishly through the digestive tract, taking an average of 77 hours to transit the system. That means that chemicals known to cause cancer in laboratory animals have nearly three full days in which to act on the vulnerable lining of the bowel. (Fiber in the diet seems to assist in moving the bile acids and cholesterol from the intestines.)

Scientists are also investigating a substance called *malonaldehyde,* produced when air breaks down certain fats. When applied to the skin of laboratory animals it can cause cancer. The substance is found in many meats (beef has the highest apparent levels of it) and the chemical process by which it is produced is encouraged by warm temperatures. The result may be an odd and hidden danger: as meat is cooked, levels of this carcinogen go up. In one study, for example, an uncooked sirloin tip roast contained only 9.5 mg of malonaldehyde per gram of meat. After cooking, the level jumped nearly 300 percent. The housewife is thus faced with a baffling paradox: while killing disease germs and parasites present in raw meat she may be producing a cancer-causing chemical that thrives on the cooking process. More research needs to be done, but the caution flag is definitely hoisted.

Another problem, found with beef in particular, is the fact that it is so often charcoal broiled. Benzopyrene, a carcinogen linked to stomach tumors and to leukemia, results when the fat of meat is charcoal broiled. In 2.2 pounds of charcoal-broiled steak there is as much benzopyrene as one would get in the smoke from 600 cigarettes!

Researchers now link meat and cancer in other ways:

1. Recent studies demonstrate that meat protein increases phenol in the urine and ammonia in the intestines. It is suggested that these may be carcinogens.
2. Some scientists believe that the cholesterol in meat may be the major agent in causation of colon cancer.
3. Epidemiological studies correlate lymph gland cancer with use of beef.
4. A high protein intake is thought to reduce immunity to cancer.

Breast cancer also seems directly related to a woman's intake of animal fat. Notice the death rate from the disease in various countries, shown in Figure 4. As the intake of animal fat and animal protein goes up, the breast cancer mortality rate goes up in an almost straight line. Table 10 shows an equally interesting relationship between the risk of breast cancer and the use of meat, eggs, and butterfat. Of the three foods, meat causes the cancer rate to rise most sharply. A study was done comparing the breast cancer rates of women graduates from Loma Linda University with those of another medical school. The women from Loma Linda had only *one-third* the breast cancer rate of those from the other university, where meat was a routine part of the diet. (Loma Linda does not serve meat in its cafeteria.)

As we have already pointed out, one of the interesting effects of the early Adventist health program was a reduction of dietary fat, especially saturated fat. One of the single greatest sources of saturated fat is meat.

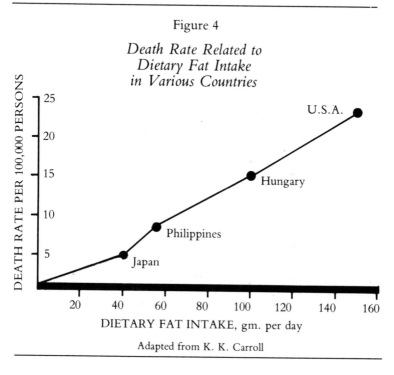

Figure 4

Death Rate Related to Dietary Fat Intake in Various Countries

Adapted from K. K. Carroll

Table 10

Relative Risk of Breast Cancer

	Meat	Eggs	Butter/Cheese
Less than 1x/Week	1.00	1.00	1.00
2–4x/Week	2.55	1.91	3.23
Almost Daily	3.83	2.86	2.10

One of the most fascinating theories to emerge from recent cancer research suggests that meat may actually lessen the body's resistance to cancer in general. To understand it you need to know a little of how the body works to fight off disease.

The most important line of defense against illness is not the red line on the floor that marks the sterile limits of the operating room. It is instead the body's own immunity, its ability to fight back. Each day we probably encounter dozens of health hazards, from the common cold to various forms of cancer. If we have eaten unwisely, stayed up too late, or depressed our white blood cell activity with too much sugar, we quickly learn that the body's defenses are not limitless. Recently scientists have suggested that saturated fat may be one of the most dangerous enemies we have, because it may actually weaken the cell membrane, the body's last major line of defense. Here is how their thinking goes.

Living tissue is composed of cells, each a complete structure of great complexity. This is the basic building block of life. The cell is surrounded by a membranous covering called the plasma membrane, a transparent structure that holds the cell together, within which all cell functions take place. When that structure is working properly, chemicals can pass in and out, nourishing the cell and removing waste products. The membrane may be porous enough to allow the proper substances to pass, but tight enough to keep out harmful ones such as viruses. Some researchers now feel that saturated fat may make that membrane more porous, thus allowing a virus to enter and to transform the cell into a wild, fast-growing outlaw called cancer. (One study showed a chemical change in the cell when beef tallow was used rather than corn oil.)

This is only a theory, admittedly. But if it turns out to be correct it could help to explain how diet and disease are linked.

Disease in general. Adventists are also concerned that other diseases in animals may pose a health threat to humans. They warn that "disease among animals is becoming more and more common, and our only safety now is in leaving meat entirely alone."[14] Recent events have proved that concern to be almost tragically well founded. Most Californians can remember a government order requiring hundreds of thousands of chickens to be killed because of highly contagious disease. And as this book is written, people in the

Midwest are being told that commercially packed turkey sold in their area somehow was contaminated with a powerful cancer-causing drug—a warning given weeks after the meat was sold and eaten. Seventy-five years ago, Adventists first raised the warning that cattle feed lot practices posed a hidden threat: "Some of the processes of fattening them for market produce disease."[15]

Adventists especially condemn pork. Even those who eat meat will usually not eat pork or any pork product. Nor will they usually eat shellfish or any other form of scavenger. "Pork," they advise, "although one of the most common articles of diet, is one of the most injurious."

Most careful Adventists also avoid fish, for the reason that fish may be "contaminated by the filth on which they feed. . . . This is especially the case where the fish come in contact with the sewage of large cities." The result? "They bring disease and death on those who do not suspect the danger."[16] A study was done on fish caught in the streams of the Fox River basin near Chicago. They had four times as many tumors as did fish caught in the clearer waters of Canada. Recently San Francisco residents have been warned about dangerously high parasite levels in striped bass caught in San Francisco Bay. If eaten, these can cause abscesses in human beings.

Long ago Adventists were cautioned that when diseased meat is eaten it "plants the seeds of disease in our own tissue," thus reducing our resistance to disease.[17] That statement is close to being vindicated by research. Several researchers now feel that our high-animal protein diet may overload and excessively stimulate the body's immune system, since it is continually being forced to react to foreign bacteria and other matter. Thus, when faced with the challenge of disease, it is less able to respond. If that theory proves correct, then Adventist concern over the link between meat and general disease will prove to be scientifically well founded.

CHEESE

As early as 1868 Adventists were advised that "cheese should never be introduced into the stomach."[18] Later cautions, in even stronger terms, pronounced it "wholly unfit for food."[19] For years scientists have been puzzling over these statements, wondering what prompted them and whether they have present validity. Some people have suggested that the advice predated pasteurization and thus was directed at the diseases commonly carried by milk in those days. Others suggest a link between the butterfat in cheese and heart disease—a consideration that merits concern and has prompted a whole new generation of "low-fat" cheeses. But do these answers really deal with the early Adventist concerns? Perhaps—and then again, perhaps not.

We'll talk more about food molds and their hazards in the next chapter. But for now we'll just say that some food molds have been associated with diseases as serious as liver cancer. Is there a possibility that the molds in cheeses may fit into this category? Research still has not told us. We do know that tyramine, a substance in certain cheeses, can elevate blood pressure in some sensitive people, producing hypertension, headaches, and associated distress. Much remains to be done before we really understand the present effect of cheese in the diet. And in the meantime, Adventists who carefully follow their health program will probably continue avoiding cheese, thereby possibly reaping health benefits research has still not uncovered.

Predictably, innovative Adventist cooks have come up with some tasty cheese substitutes using soy derivatives, polyunsaturated oils, and herb seasonings. Some of them (such as pimento stuffing for celery) taste so close to the real thing that it is difficult to tell the difference. Other varieties are used as toppings for stuffed peppers, "pizza steaks," and a variety of other interesting vegetarian recipes. We've included some of these cheese substitutes in the Appendix.

SUMMARY

We have talked about some of the more unique aspects of the Adventist dietary program. We have seen that there are some foods, eaten by most people, that Adventists avoid. We have also seen that for each such item they have specific reasons, often supported by recent scientific research.

By now you probably have a question that you would like answered: what *do* they eat?

It is time to talk about that.

Chapter 3

How to Cook and How to Eat

Sometime try asking an Adventist, "What *do* you eat?" He will probably respond at first with an incredulous stare, as though your question makes no sense at all. So far as Adventists are concerned they eat everything—with a few conspicuous exceptions. The exceptions? Excess sugar. Meat, usually. Highly spiced foods. Alcohol. Stimulants, such as tea and coffee. Beyond that, the sky is the limit. There are many varieties of grain in the world, scores of varieties of fruit. Nuts and vegetables are in such abundance that one could never hope to get bored with repetition. Replacing meat in the diet is a challenge most Adventist cooks accept with gusto. They are prolific writers of cookbooks. They frequently conduct cooking classes, open to the public, to share their new ideas on nutrition. They produce commercial meat substitutes and other foods, available at most large markets, and their Sanitarium brand food industry absolutely dominates the breakfast cereal market in Australasia.

And so, sometime, just for fun, ask an Adventist what he or she *does* eat. You may get more than you bargained for. In the meantime, we will answer much of that question here. Read with an open mind, and be willing to try an idea or two. Your benefits will probably be greater longevity, less risk of major diseases, and—purely as a bonus—a lower food bill.

FRUITS, NUTS, AND GRAINS

"In grains, fruits, vegetables, and nuts are to be found all the food elements that we need."

"Grains, fruits, nuts, and vegetables . . . prepared in as simple and natural a manner as possible, are the most healthful and nourishing. They impart a strength, a power of endurance, and a vigor of

37

intellect, that are not afforded by a more complex and stimulating diet."[1]

These are two landmark Adventist statements on diet. This is the premise from which much of their dietary program proceeds. Is the premise valid?

Think about their recommended diet for a moment and you will realize that it is high in carbohydrates. Today Americans get only about 22 percent of their calories in the form of complex carbohydrates. According to the Senate Select Committee on Nutrition and Human Needs, that figure ought to be doubled. In other words, we need to be getting nearly half our calories from complex carbohydrates—a goal that is difficult to reach with a diet heavily weighted in favor of meat. (Meat is a unique food in that it contains little or no carbohydrate.)

In America, consumption of carbohydrates has dropped significantly since World War II. We now consume nearly 25 percent less complex carbohydrates than Americans did in 1909. Many scientists are beginning to wonder if this may help to explain our high rate of heart disease. In 1976 Drs. William and Sonja Connor pointed out that "most population groups with a low incidence of coronary heart disease consume from 65 percent to 85 percent of their total energy in the form of carbohydrates derived from whole grains (cereals) and tubers (potatoes)."[2]

Dr. Jeremiah Stamler reports lower cholesterol levels in those Europeans who eat a high proportion of carbohydrates. (Interestingly, when these same population groups emigrate to the United States and adopt the typical American diet, their blood cholesterol levels rise to the higher levels prevalent among Americans.)

The conclusion? "High-carbohydrate diets are quite appropriate for both normal individuals and for most of those with hyperlipidemia (high levels of fat in the blood), provided that the *carbohydrate is largely derived from grains and tubers,* and that the person stays within the limits for normal weight" [italics added].[3]

The Connors also report that a high-complex carbohydrate diet is important in the treatment of diabetics, because it reduces hazards often associated with diabetes. They note that on a high-complex carbohydrate diet some diabetics tolerate glucose better, while others enjoy better stability in their need for insulin.

Finally, the Senate Select Committee on Nutrition and Human Needs advocates the high-carbohydrate diet for a number of other reasons. It affords more natural fiber, important in preventing many diseases. It provides vitamins and minerals, and lastly, purely as a bonus, it enables a person to control weight more easily since "the high water content and bulk of fruits and vegetables and bulk of whole grain can bring satisfaction of appetite more quickly than do foods high in fat and sugar."[4]

We have discussed many advantages of a high-complex carbohydrate diet, recognized as such not only by Adventists but by noted scientific researchers. Are there corresponding problems associated with a low-carbohydrate diet? The answer is *yes*.

A low-carbohydrate diet is undesirable because it actually lessens one's power of endurance. Scientists have known this for many years: as early as the 1920s a study was done comparing the endurance of vegetarians with that of meat eaters. As strange as it may sound to our conditioned ears, the vegetarians' exercise endurance was nearly *twice* that of those who ate meat. Moreover, the vegetarians recovered from fatigue much more rapidly. Recently a Swedish scientist repeated that experiment. Athletes on a high-meat diet, high in fat and protein, were compared with athletes eating mainly grains and vegetables. On a rigorous endurance test, the group on a highly vegetarian diet lasted nearly *three times* longer than those on the meat diet.

Are all the food elements we need really found in a vegetarian diet? What about vitamin B_{12}, vitamin D, vitamin A? Before we knew that carotene in carrots and many other foods produces vitamin A in the body, people thought that animal products were necessary in order to get it. Now we know that they aren't. We know that vitamin D can be had from the action of sunshine on the skin. As to vitamin B^{12}, there is still some uncertainty, although there is a possibility that it may be produced by intestinal bacteria. It is a substance added to so many foods that it is becoming more and more difficult to find a person nutritionally deficient in B_{12}. Nevertheless persons who choose a "vegan" or total vegetarian diet are advised by many nutritionists to supplement their diet in order to be sure of getting this vitamin.

Now reflect on the statement that grains, fruits, nuts, and vegetables "impart a strength, a power of endurance . . . not afforded by a more complex and stimulating diet." Once again, the premise seems scientifically sound.

How, then, does one go about using these foods?

Fruits. One of the greatest advantages of fruit is that it is usually ready to eat, right from nature. It needs very little preparation and virtually no additives such as sugar or salt. It can thus be enjoyed in large amounts by nearly everybody, including most heart patients, hypertensives, and all but some diabetics and hypoglycemics. It does not require cooking, and therefore retains vitamin C and other substances that are broken down by heat and oxidation. It is extremely low in fat, with a very few exceptions, such as olives and avocados.

And it is eye appealing. Sometime, just for an experiment, take three or four varieties of fruit and dice them into small cubes. Try to use fruits of contrasting colors. Place alternating layers of fruit in tall parfait glasses, using various combinations. The result will be one of the most attractive desserts you can imagine. In our hospital health education programs we frequently do this very demonstration, calling men out of the audience to create these dessert dishes. Many of them have never used a serving spoon in their lives, and usually humor gives way to delighted surprise when the audience sees that even men can create beautiful desserts using only fruit in its natural state. This is an excellent way to attract children to fruit instead of to refined sweets.

Another way to use fruit, particularly with children, is in juices. Many fruits combine nicely to form colorful juices that attract children by sight as well as by taste. Our hospital health education team is frequently asked to conduct public school health days. Since youngsters often use soft drinks in excess, we always include a demonstration or two of fruit juices, done with a blender right in front of the students. There are almost limitless combinations, but for starters we usually do two: orange juice and banana, and a combination of pineapple juice, peaches, bananas, and strawberries. The color is striking (and is free from Red Dye No. 2), and the taste usually brings even skeptical high school students back for seconds.

For someone with an incurable sweet tooth, fruit is an ideal substitute for refined sugar. Recognizing that many people enjoy their breakfast pastries and dinner desserts, Adventists have devised a number of recipes that use only natural fruit for sweetening: apple pie, banana cream pie, bear claws, cookies, and a delicious date bar, to name a few. Just to give you a feel for what we are talking about, we have included a few such recipes in the Appendix. To really explore sugar substitutes you may want to go to one of the cookbooks listed in the Appendix.

What medical benefits can you expect from switching to fruit instead of sugar?

The obvious, of course, is lessened tooth decay. Another advantage is a possible reduction of your risk of diabetes. In countries where more than 10 percent of the calories are taken as sugar, there is a high incidence of diabetes. In the United States we consume 17 percent of our calories as sugar.

But what about heart disease? In the bloodstream are fats known as *triglycerides.* Researchers are still puzzling over all that they do in the body, but many scientists—particularly those in Europe—feel that they are related to heart disease. We know that in women over fifty, triglyceride levels bear a significant relationship to risk of heart attack. There is a possibility that triglycerides may cause cholesterol to be deposited more rapidly in the arteries, thus accelerating the onset of cardiovascular disease. Refined sugar tends to raise triglyceride levels. Fruit, with its natural sugar, usually does not. There are some scientists who do not believe that sugar elevates blood triglycerides. But in the thousands of people who have gone through our hospital coronary risk evaluation, those with high blood triglycerides have come back to normal when sugar, ice cream, and other sweets were eliminated from the diet.

Do Adventists offer any cautions on the use of fruit? Just one. Be sure that it is "absolutely free from decay."[5] There is more to this warning than a statement of the obvious. We are now learning that some foods, if not picked and used when fresh, can develop molds that contain powerful carcinogens. For example, apples can develop a mold that contains *patulin,* a substance known to produce liver cancer in laboratory mice. Many years ago, long before scientists really understood the significance of decay in food, Adventists were cautioned that "if people could see what the microscope reveals in regard to the cider they buy, few would be willing to drink it. Often those who manufacture cider for the market are not careful as to the condition of the fruit used, and the juice of wormy and decayed apples is expressed. . . . This pleasant beverage is wholly unfit for human use."[6]

Are Adventists condemning apples or apple juice? No. They merely urge that apples, as well as other food, "should be carefully gathered and preserved."[7] For this reason many Adventists are enthusiastic about growing their own food. For people in urban areas this is often impossible, but many Adventists relish the discipline of country life, together with the security that comes from fresh, untainted produce. More and more Americans are coming to share that enthusiasm.

Finally, they believe that fruit can have medicinal value. Its fiber content promotes healthy digestion, while the vitamins in fresh fruit may often help ward off annoyances such as the common cold. Olives in particular are considered useful in relieving gastric irritation. To quote one of their statements: "Olives may be so prepared as to be eaten with good results at every meal."[8]

Nuts. Adventists see nuts as an extremely useful substitute for the protein found in meat. Nuts offer many advantages. They are tasty. They have a relatively long shelf life, which makes storage easy. The oils in nuts help to provide the satiety, or feeling of "fullness," which one gets from eating meat. Like fruit, they require little in the way of preparation. Some of them, such as walnuts and almonds, can be eaten raw. At most, nuts require only a little roasting. And if one wishes to go further and use them as part of a main entrée, they provide high-quality protein relatively low in saturated fat.

Adventists have experimented with nuts for a hundred years, and the result is a large collection of entrée recipes using them instead of meat. Combined with grains, vegetables, and seasonings, they can be made into some really exotic low-saturated fat, cholesterol-free main dishes. To give you an idea of what can be done, we have included in the Appendix a few of the more interesting recipes Adventist cooks use in preparing nut dishes.

Cautions regarding the use of nuts? Yes, just one: don't overdo it. Nuts do have a high oil content that is far less saturated than animal fat but should not be used in unlimited quantities. To quote the Adventists, "If they were used more sparingly by some, the results would be more satisfactory. . . . Almonds are preferable to peanuts; but peanuts, in limited quantities, may be used in connection with grains to make nourishing and digestible food."[9]

One Adventist writing suggests that the proportion of nuts in a dish be limited to about 10 to 15 percent. One can only assume that this would optimize their usefulness without including excess amounts of fat.

For those who do not wish to take the time necessary to prepare the dishes shown in the Appendix, Adventists have devised commercial meat substitutes using nuts and grains. They are readily available at large markets and can often be cooked just as they come from the can—although most serious Adventist cooks would urge you to dress them up with sauces and trimmings rather than to merely heat and eat.

Grains. "There is more religion in a good loaf of bread than many think."[10]

With that practical statement, Adventists approach the whole concept of using grains in the diet. They have long stressed the importance of good, whole grain bread—not limited to wheat flour, but using a variety of grains so as to get the benefits each has to offer. In recent years we have seen these products blossom on supermarket shelves as the idea of health catches on in America, but Adventists have been urging whole grain and multigrain breads since before the turn of the century.

Bread, however, is not the only use to which they put grains. They also use them in many entrée dishes, some of them quite exotic. (For example, try a recipe called "Ala Pilaf," shown in the Appendix.) According to a spokesman for the Department of Agriculture, there are literally dozens of available grain varieties in the United States alone, an assortment that gives the resourceful cook quite a selection to choose from. Adventist grain dishes range all the way from simple boiled wheat (a robust and surprisingly tasty breakfast food) to highly complex dishes that demand the best that a good cook has to offer.

People are often surprised to learn that grains contain sufficient protein to replace meat as a main dish. Actually, that is not surprising when one stops to think about it, because beef—one of America's favorite protein foods—is most prized when fattened on grain. The protein content of grain can be processed so as to exceed that of most meats. Loma Linda Foods, an Adventist health food manufacturer, produces meat substitutes from grain that have more protein per calorie than chicken, veal, hamburger, and many other meats. Even plain whole wheat bread delivers 16 percent of its calories as protein—a level one-and-a-half times the Food and Nutrition Board's Recommended Daily Allowance.

Table 11

Protein Foods

Grams Protein Per Serving

	Size Portion	Grams
Chicken leg	5 ounces	29.1
Beef steak, porterhouse	3 ounces	23.0
Salmon, canned	3 ounces	22.1
Kidney beans	1 cup	19.6
Vegeburger	1/2 cup	19.0
Dinner cuts	2	16.6
Cottage cheese	1/3 cup	14.6
Eggs	2	13.8
Beef liver, fried	2 ounces	13.5
Granola	1 cup	10.9
Peanuts	1/4 cup	9.7
Wheat germ	1/2 cup	8.5
Milk	1 cup	8.5
Swiss cheese	1 ounce	7.4
Frankfurter	1	7.0
Egg	1	6.7
Clams	3 ounces	6.7
Bran flakes	1 cup	4.3
Corn	1 ear	3.7
Ice cream	1 slice	3.2
Brewer's yeast	1 tablespoon	3.0
Baked potato	1 medium	2.4
Whole wheat bread	1 1/2 slices	2.1
Almonds	11	1.5
Rice	1 cup	4.2
Asparagus	1 cup	4.2
Linkett	1	7.4
Soy milk	1 cup	7.3
Dinner round	1	8.0

Perhaps this is a good point at which to talk about protein. For years we have been urged to eat massive quantities of it, until many people have come to believe that it should be the main element of the

Table 12
Protein Foods

Percentage of Calories as Protein in Common Foods

Cottage cheese—skim milk	84
creamed	55
Dinner cuts (an Adventist meat substitute)	77
Vegeburger (an Adventist meat substitute)	68
Chicken breast	68
Veal chuck, thin	61
Yeast	58
Beef liver, fried	49
Beef round	47
Salmon, canned	46
Chicken broiler, fried	42
Beef hamburger	35–53
Buttermilk	42
Linketts (meat substitute)	41
Dinner rounds (meat substitute)	38
Tofu	38
Eggs	35
Swiss cheese	32
Broccoli	29
Beefsteak	23–33
Asparagus	27
Pork loin	24–30
Lentils	25
Whole milk	23
Kidney beans	23
Bacon	21
Peanuts	16
Whole wheat bread	16
Angel food cake	13
Corn	10
Almonds	9
Baked potato	8
Rice	7
Bran flakes	6
Ice cream	5

diet. Admittedly, it is important. But is it possible to get too much? And if so, are there any dangers?

The answer to both questions is a decided *yes*. Many years ago researchers tested laboratory animals on diets in which the protein level ranged from 10 percent to 26 percent. The result? The test animals lived the longest on a diet that contained from 10 to 14 percent protein. At 26 percent protein levels there was significant shortening of the lifespan. The animals matured more quickly and died just as quickly—sobering evidence that excess protein may speed everything up, from maturation to death. A second problem is that excess protein apparently overloads the kidneys. Test animals fed a high-protein diet over long periods of time showed kidney enlargement in every single instance. Some of them developed kid-

Table 13

Biological Value of Food Proteins★

Food Material	Biological Value %
Egg, yolk	95
Egg, whole	94
Milk, raw, liquid	90
Milk, evaporated	88
Lactalbumin	84
Milk, dried skim	84
Egg, white	83
Pork tenderloin	79
Linseed meal	78
Corn, germ	78
Beef kidney	77
Beef liver	77
Beef muscle	76
Wheat germ	75
Rice, white	75
Soybean flour	75
Pork, ham	74
Beef heart	74
Casein	73
Cheese, Swiss	73
Watermelon seed	73
Red salmon	72

Cashew	72
Sweet potato	72
Coconut	71
Sesame seed	71
Cheese, Limburger	69
Potato	67
Wheat, whole	67
Sunflower seed flour	65
Soybean curd	65
Wheat, puffed	64
Barley	64
Yeast, brewer's	63
Pumpkin seed	63
Cottonseed flour	62
Alfalfa leaf	61
Pecan	60
Corn, whole	60
Soybeans, raw	59
Rye	58
Mung beans	58
Kaoliang	56
Millet	56
Wheat bread, 100% extraction	56
Peanut, roasted	56
English walnut	56
Brazil nut	54
Wheat bread, 80% extraction	54
Hegari	53
Wheat bread, 85% extraction	53
White flour	52
Almond	51
Wheat bread, 70% extraction	51
Filbert	50
White bread, 6% milk solids	50
Peas, raw	48
White bread, 2% milk solids	48
Tankage	48
White bread, no milk	45
Navy beans, cooked	38
Cocoa	37

*From *Proteins and Amino Acids in Nutrition* (New York: Rhinhold, 1948), by Melville Sahyun, p. 60, 61.

ney disease. Too much protein seems to overwork the body in general. Unlike fat, it cannot be stored in the body, and hence excess amounts must be converted into carbohydrates and fats—an additional demand placed on the liver.

In an earlier section, we have already seen that some researchers fear that our high-animal protein diet may weaken the body's resistance to disease by overloading the immune system. In 1959 a researcher reported that when animals were given a high-calorie, high-protein diet, there was a doubling in the incidence of tumors.

Is it possible that in still another instance the Adventists have been right all along? Notice that the diet that they recommend automatically provides protein in the 10 percent range—exactly the level at which animal studies show optimum lifespan. Scientists can argue for years over whether such studies really apply to human beings, but there is one fact they can't debate: Adventist men age 35–40 live 6.2 years longer than do their non-Adventist counterparts.

Take a look at table 14. If a person receives one-third of his or her calories from fruits, one-third from grains or potatoes, and one-third from legumes or greens, the result would be a diet with 13 percent of

---

Table 14

A. Protein Content of Food Groups as a Percentage of Calories

Fruits	3.7	Milk, whole	22.0
Potatoes	6.7	Milk, skim, dry	42.7
Rice	7.1	Eggs, fresh	33.3
Corn	10.0	Cheese, hard	42.6
Wheat flour		Salmon, canned	49.9
(medium extraction)	13.0	Tuna, canned (low fat)	95.0
Beans, peas, dry	22.3	Chicken	25.5
Cabbage, fresh	24.4	Beef	27.4
		Pork	13.9

B. Minimal Protein Needs

With one-third of calories from fruits, one-third from grains or potatoes, and one-third from legumes or greens, one would have 13 percent of his calories as protein, which equals the Recommended Dietary Allowance, which is twice minimum needs.

the calories as protein. This exceeds the published Recommended Dietary Allowance, which in turn is *twice* what scientists consider our absolute minimum need. Faced with this data, responsible scientists now say that if people eat sufficient fruits, grains, nuts, and vegetables to maintain their ideal weight, it is virtually impossible to get too little protein. Compare that conclusion with the Adventist statement from 1906: "In grains, fruits, vegetables, and nuts are to be found all the food elements that we need."[11]

There is a hidden bonus to this program that becomes rapidly apparent at the grocery check-out stand. Notice the data on table 15, showing the comparative cost of protein from vegetable sources as opposed to that from meat. In today's economy, those differences have a persuasion quite apart from nutrition.

Table 15
Comparison of Animal vs. Vegetable Proteins

	Per 100 Grams		Per 100 Calories	
	Round steak	Kidney beans	Round steak	Kidney beans
Cost in cents	27.9	1.8	10.7	2.0
Calories	261.0	90.0	100.0	100.0
Grams	100.0	100.0	38.0	111.0
Protein, gms	28.6	5.7	12.5	6.3
Calcium, mg	130.0	40.0	4.0	44.0
Phosphorus, mg	250.0	124.0	96.0	136.0
Iron, mg	3.5	1.9	1.45	2.1
Vitamin A, IU	3.0	0	0	0
Vitamin B_1, mh	0.08	0.05	0.03	0.05
Riboflavin, mg	0.22	0.05	0.1	0.05
Niacin, mg	5.6	0.8	2.35	0.9
Vitamin C, mg	0	0	0	0
Fat, gm	14.5	0.4	5.5	0.4
% Fat calories	47.3	3.4	47.3	3.4
P/S ratio	0.06	—	0.06	—
CHO, gm	0	20.0	0	18.0

Is it necessary to have a complete protein at each meal? Years ago, following certain animal studies, scientists thought so. Rats fed half of the essential amino acids in one meal and the other half at subsequent meals had poor growth. Other animals were fed all the essential amino acids except one—either lysine or methionine—which was fed to them separately twelve hours later. Again, there was poor growth. Because of these studies (done between 1929 and 1950), it was thought that people should eat a complete protein at each meal.

But the studies really mean little in the real world, because no foods (except gelatin and protein isolates) are totally lacking in a specific amino acid. More recent studies show that enzymes from intestinal juices supply amino acids. In one study rats were fed wheat, which is low in lysine. Supplemented lysine was given to them twelve hours later. No difference could be detected when they were compared with rats given lysine at the time they were fed the wheat. It is now apparent that there is no validity to the old concern about getting a complete protein at every meal.

Table 16

Nutrients Lost in the Refining Process of Whole Wheat

	% Loss*
Vitamin B₁ (thiamine)	86
Vitamin B₂ (riboflavin)	70
Niacin	86
Iron	84
Vitamin B₆ (pyridoxine)	60
Folic acid	70
Pantothenic acid	54
Biotin	90
Calcium	50
Phosphorus	78
Copper	75
Magnesium	72
Manganese	71

*Only vitamins B₁, B₂, niacin and the mineral iron are added back in the enrichment process. Calculated from "Lesser Known Vitamins in Foods," *J Am Diet Assn* 38: 240–243, 1961, as compiled by Mervyn G. Hardinge and Hulda Crooks.

Here are the three basic rules Adventists follow when using grains:

Use whole grains. Remember that all of the advantages listed above pertain to *whole* grains, not refined flour. Adventists believe that "fine flour bread cannot impart to the system the nourishment that you will find in the unbolted-wheat bread. The common use of bolted-wheat bread cannot keep the system in a healthy condition."[12] ("Unbolted" refers to coarser, whole grain flour.) The profound implications of that statement come into focus in table 16. Notice that when wheat is refined it loses up to 86 percent of such vital elements as vitamin B1. Additionally, whole grains are an important source of fiber. No wonder Adventists are advised to use the natural product. (They often joke about the term *enriched* flour. It is enriched, they say, in the same way you would be enriched if a thief took your wallet with $10 in it and gave you back 60¢ for bus fare to get home.)

Table 17

Comparison of Three B Vitamins and Iron in Pound Loaves of Wheat Bread[1]

Wheat Bread (2% Nonfat Dry Milk)	Thiamine mg	Riboflavin mg	Niacin mg	Iron mg
Unenriched	0.40	0.36	5.6	3.2
Enriched[2]	1.13	0.77	10.4	10.9
Whole wheat	1.17	0.56	12.9	10.4

[1]U.S. Department of Agriculture: Handbook No. 8.
[2]May furnish as an optional ingredient vitamin D to make up 150–750 U.S.P. units per pound loaf.
May also contain added calcium salts (including milk solids) so that the total is 300–800 mg calcium per pound loaf.

Use a variety of grains. "All wheat flour is not best for a continuous diet. A mixture of wheat, oatmeal, and rye would be more nutritious."[13] Fortunately, mixed grain breads are now becoming readily available so that the general public can get the benefit of something that used to be difficult to find. Another way to get variety is to try a breakfast of whole wheat and rye toast with cooked oatmeal.

When making bread, do it right: There are a number of Adventist suggestions for good, wholesome bread.

Use sweet rather than sour dough. In bread, as in other foods, freshness and freedom from decay are important to Adventist cooks.

Avoid the use of baking powder or soda. Adventists believe that these are harmful in the stomach and often cause difficulties throughout the system. Soda is known to destroy thiamin, an essential vitamin.

Make bread in small loaves rather than large ones. The reason for this is quite interesting. Live yeast in the digestive tract depletes the body of vitamin B1. When bread is cooked in smaller loaves, the yeast in the interior of the loaf is more apt to be killed by the heat, thus avoiding this problem.

For the same general reason given above, avoid eating fresh bread hot from the oven. (Perhaps this is the hardest rule to follow!) Adventists believe it to be more difficult to digest than bread that has cooled and dried out somewhat. Additionally, there is the danger of live yeast causing vitamin deficiency if bread is eaten while still hot and moist.

Use toasted bread. The old German standby, zwieback, is strongly recommended. This hearty food, similar to the melba toast given to young children, is thoroughly dry. It can be made by cutting slices of fresh bread and toasting them or heating them in a warm oven. It has an added advantage in that it keeps much longer than fresh bread. Adventists often eat this with fruit in the evening instead of eating a heavy evening meal. They believe that by eating a light meal one gets better rest at night and is more ready to eat a hearty breakfast in the morning.

Incidentally, Adventists also believe that hard foods such as dried bread are preferable to soft foods. The reason is that they have to be chewed thoroughly. The digestive process begins in the mouth, and one loses some of the value from food when it is swallowed whole — or washed down with liquids. We'll talk more about liquids with meals shortly.

Biscuits are generally avoided because they are served hot, and because they contain baking soda or powder—two principles we talked about earlier.

Avoid using milk in the bread dough. Bread made with water will keep longer and is preferred by Adventist cooks. (Milk in commercially baked bread requires more chemical preservatives.)

A series of highly restrictive rules? Perhaps. But remember that they are really just suggestions, each based on a physiological reason, which the individual is free to follow or to ignore. And the fact that they exist shows the importance that Adventists attach to good bread.

LEGUMES

Beans, lentils, and other legumes are another Adventist answer to meat. They are easily prepared and are extremely inexpensive. Note the cost comparisons in table 15 showing the relative cost per unit of protein. Few articles of food offer as good a buy. Beans and other legumes are an important source of fiber. They also offer other benefits. Beans are known to lower cholesterol. (One famed nutritionist wrote a whole book on beans because of their importance in lowering blood cholesterol levels.) Another benefit is fewer calories. One cup of beans has only 250 calories; six ounces of steak has 660 calories—a good example of how the use of meat, as a high-density food, makes it more difficult to control one's weight.

In the Appendix we have listed a few interesting legume recipes, showing how these versatile foods can even be baked into casserole dishes that take the place of meat loaf.

VEGETABLES

Perhaps this simple statement, taken from Adventist health writings, says it best: "All should be acquainted with the special value of fruits and vegetables fresh from the orchard and garden."[14]

Vegetables offer a special advantage to anyone with a few square feet of unused soil: they can be grown in one's own garden and thus offer the treat of having something on the table that is absolutely fresh. With the discovery of carcinogens in certain plant molds, scientists are beginning to understand the importance Adventists have long attached to getting food free from the "slightest sign of decay."[15] The very best way to get this, of course, is right from your own garden.

Fresh vegetables offer the obvious advantage of supplying vitamins, minerals, and trace elements at low cost. Americans spend millions of dollars each year for expensive food supplements that cannot improve on the nutrients available in fresh garden produce.

Here are the Adventist suggestions for using vegetables:

Get them fresh and absolutely free from decay. This can be a tall order when vegetables are purchased off the grocer's shelf, but careful shopping will help. If you can, plant a garden. If not, then find produce stands with field-fresh merchandise. Use only produce that is "sound and unaffected by any disease or decay."[16]

Use a good variety, for appetite's sake as well as for nutrition. One of the cardinal points of Adventist dietary doctrine is that food should be enjoyed. They believe that "it is a religious duty ... to prepare healthful food in different ways, so that it may be eaten with enjoyment."[17] The bonus, of course, is a variety of nutrients from the different foods, thus assuring a balanced, economical diet.

Avoid combining fruits and vegetables. Adventists believe that it is best not to combine fruits and vegetables at the same meal. This may sound like a strange, rather arbitrary idea, but they have reasons for it. "If the digestion is feeble, the use of both will often cause distress, and inability to put forth mental effort."[18] Here one sees the link, so often described in Adventist writings, between the brain and the stomach. In many ways medical science recognizes that link—aggravation of ulcers, for example, when one is under stress—but Adventists carry it to a very high level. The concept of wholeness is very much a part of all their teaching, and this is one good example of that.

How does one get around the problem of combining fruits and vegetables? Many careful Adventist health reformers do so by making their largest meal breakfast, on the theory that they need the greatest intake of food at the start of the work day. Lunch is also a robust meal, at which vegetables are often served. Fruit is taken in the evening, perhaps with bread or some other grain product. It is a light meal, taken as early as possible to avoid sleeping on a full stomach. Thus, vegetables are segregated to one meal, usually in midday, and fruit is taken either in the morning or at night. There is nothing difficult about the plan; it merely requires a little thought ahead of time.

"It is the variety and mixture of meat, vegetables, fruit, wines, tea, coffee, sweet cakes, and rich pies that ruin the stomach," Adventists have been told,[19] and that advice even goes for too many varieties of the best food if taken at one sitting. Usually they will try to limit the varieties of food to just a few, serve those in quantities adequate to send everyone away from the table happy, and wait until the next meal for further variety in the diet. They feel that following that rule will bring a quieter stomach, a clearer mind, and a happier disposition.

Use vegetables as an aid to weight reduction. If individuals are concerned about calories, vegetables can be their greatest allies. In table 18 we have shown how many servings of various vegetables one would have to eat to reach a diet of only 510 calories. It is a staggering total, literally more than the most commodious stomach could hope to hold. The lesson? You *can* eat all you want to and still lose weight. Simply choose your food wisely.

Table 18

Nutrient Content of Selected Vegetables and Fruits

Nutrients	Amounts in Vegetables[1]	Amounts in Fruits[2]
Protein	30 gm	30 gm
Calcium	868 mg	270 gm
Iron	12.8 mg	15 mg
Vitamin A	74,840 I.U.	39,600 I.U.
Thiamine	1.46 mg	0.6 mg
Riboflavin	2.06 mg	1.5 mg
Niacin	17.8 mg	30 mg
Vitamin C	276 mg	210 mg

[1]Includes 2 cups grated carrots, 6 cups string beans, and 8 cups summer squash, a total of 510 calories. This meets the recommended daily allowance for calcium, vitamin A, thiamine, riboflavin, and vitamin C, as well as niacin, for all practical purposes. It also meets the male RDA for iron.
[2]This includes 30 peaches, with 1050 calories. It meets the RDA for iron for men, for vitamin A, thiamine, niacin, and vitamin C, as well as the riboflavin requirement for women.

HOW TO COOK

By now it should come as no surprise that Adventists have many suggestions on the most healthful ways to cook. We have already touched on a few. Here they are, given together:

Recognize the importance of good cooking. Adventists consider cooking to be one of the most important jobs in the world. "The one who understands the art of properly preparing food . . . is worthy of higher commendation than those engaged in any other line of work."[20] Perhaps this philosophy is the reason so many Adventist women take pleasure in conducting public cooking schools.

Recognize that good cooking is a science that requires careful study and preparation. "Skill must be united with simplicity. To do this, women must read, and then patiently reduce what they read to practice. . . . Learn how to cook with simplicity, and yet in a manner to secure the most palatable and healthful food."[21] Repeatedly, Adventist writings stress the need to understand the principles of diet and physiology so that cooking can be done in the way best suited to the human system. Books on this subject are listed in the Appendix.

As far as possible, cook with simplicity. Adventists firmly believe that too many varieties of even the best food at one meal make digestion more difficult, overstress the system, and cause repercussions such as loss of mental acuity. At the same time, they demand that food be inspiring to the appetite. "The serving of a great variety of dishes absorbs time, money, and taxing labor, without accomplishing any good."[22] Instead, Adventist cooks are urged to put their effort into fewer dishes, make them highly appetizing, and serve them in such a pleasant, happy atmosphere that mealtime will become one of the high points of the day. If food is not enjoyed, they reason, "the body will not be so well nourished."[23] Thus, while there is less variety at any one meal, more effort is put into making the dishes that are served highly appetizing.

Careful Adventists avoid spices, condiments, and other foods that tend to irritate the lining of the stomach. For people who are used to a highly spiced diet, their menus may seem a litte bland (although skillful Adventist cooks can do much to overcome that with nonir- ritating herb seasonings). But there is sound scientific evidence that their caution is well founded. The best example is the diet used by ulcer patients. It can be difficult to cure ulcers while highly spiced foods are used. Why? Because they have such a devastating effect on the mucous lining of the stomach and duodenum.

Table 19 is a list of the more commonly used spices. Table 20 shows the herbs used by Adventist cooks to season food without those accompanying dangers.

Table 19

Know Your Condiments

Irritating, Stimulating, Harmful	Strongly Aromatic, Irritating	Slightly Irritating
Pepper, Cayenne	Cloves	Allspice
Black	Ginger	Anise
White	Paprika (Hungarian)	Cassia
Chili powder		Cinnamon
Horse-radish		Mace
Mustard		Nutmeg

Ingredients of Mixed Spices

Poultry Seasoning	Curry, Foreign Type	Curry, American Type
Allspice	Black Pepper	Cinnamon
Marjoram	Cayenne Pepper	Cloves
Nutmeg	Cinnamon	Coriander
Sage	Cloves	Ginger
Savory	Nutmeg	Mace
Thyme		Nutmeg
		Pepper
		Turmeric

Adventists have been advised to avoid pickles, mince pies, mustard, peppers, curry, and other irritating seasonings. They also avoid "rich" foods such as spicy gravies. Note the following quotation from the Adventist book, *Counsels on Diets and Foods*. The reasons behind it, and the scientific evidence which supports it, are equally fascinating.

"Luxurious dishes are placed before the children—spiced foods, rich gravies, cakes, and pastries. This highly seasoned food irritates the stomach, and *causes a craving for still stronger stimulants.*" [italics supplied]

Table 20

Sweet Herbs, Not Irritating

Bay leaf	Parsley
Caraway seed	Peppermint
Celery salt	Saffron
Chives	Sage
Dillseed	Savory
Fennel	Spearmint
Marjoram	Thyme
Mint	Turmeric
Onion salt	Wintergreen
Paprika (Spanish type, highly colored)	

Recently a research team decided to test the hypothesis in this statement. They took two groups of laboratory rats and fed them two separate diets. One was the diet recommended in Adventist writings; the other was the typical American teenager's diet, including a high proportion of meat, sugar, and junk food. Each group of rats was provided both water and alcohol to drink; which they chose was strictly up to them. The result? Rats fed a careful diet drank virtually no alcohol. Those fed the typical American teenager's diet drank alcohol in preference to water. And when coffee and spices were added to the menu (in the form of powder, mixed with their food), alcohol consumption shot up to a high level.

Use salt in moderation. Salt is a vital electrolyte, needed by the human body. But too much of it is associated with numerous problems, such as fluid retention and high blood pressure. For many years Adventists have been urged to use this substance in sensible moderation. Too much salt causes another problem. It promotes an unnatural thirst, leading to drinking large amounts of fluids with meals. We'll talk more about that shortly.

Avoid the use of grease. Lard, beef tallow, and similar greases are carefully avoided. They usually result in a high cooking temperature, thereby destroying substances such as vitamin C. They cause an increase in blood cholesterol. They slow the process of digestion. When superheated, they can produce highly carcinogenic substances such as benzopyrene.

Avoid vinegar. Many Adventists believe that vinegar seriously interferes with digestion, leading to decay of food in the bowel rather than to a healthy digestive process. As a result, some feel that both liver and kidney difficulties can result. (Vinegar is 3 to 4 percent acetic acid. In a laboratory bottle, this would be labeled as a poison!)

About the only time this presents a real problem is in salad dressings, and they have come up with some palatable alternatives. (Lemon juice offers a zesty way to perk up a salad without vinegar. Corn oil salad dressing is often used—homemade without vinegar. Another, called "zero" dressing because of its low calories, uses tomato juice and herbs. These are shown in the Appendix.)

Serve food warm rather than very cold or very hot. Perhaps one of the worst habits we Americans have fallen into is the obligatory glass of water, half-filled with crushed ice, which we are handed even before we order our food. Adventists believe that when very cold food is taken into the stomach, the whole digestive process is hindered and does not return to normal until the blood has rewarmed the chilled stomach lining. They therefore avoid extremely cold foods. Likewise, they avoid extremely hot foods because their use causes several wide-ranging problems. "The stomach is greatly injured by a large quantity of hot food and drink. Thus the throat and digestive organs, and through them the other organs of the body, are enfeebled."[24] To people accustomed to starting a meal with ice water and steaming coffee, that instruction may sound strange. But there is a great deal of common sense in it, if one stops to think it through. Recent dental studies have concluded that tooth damage may result from the sudden expansion and contraction of the teeth as they are alternately frozen and blistered, resulting in hairline cracks. Adventists also believe that "the free use of hot drinks is debilitating."[25] "Very hot food ought not to be taken into the stomach. Soups, puddings, and other articles of the kind, are often eaten too hot, and as a consequence the stomach is debilitated. Let them become partly cooled before they are eaten."[26]

Avoid adulterated food. This concern, now shared by millions of Americans, was given by the Adventists back in 1905: "We must be satisfied with pure, simple food, prepared in a simple manner.... *Adulterated substances are to be avoided*" [italics supplied].[27] Why? Because, in the Adventist understanding of health, the mind is once again intimately affected by the diet. "You should use the most simple food, prepared in the most simple manner, that the fine nerves of the brain be not weakened, benumbed, or paralyzed . . ."[28] Only today are we beginning to see how profound the results can be when food is adulterated with additives whose medical effects are not fully known. Will the other half of the Adventist warning, concerning the need for simplicity in diet, also emerge in scientific research? Time will tell.

Teach your children the joy of healthful cooking. Perhaps one of the best examples of the *why* behind Adventist health principles is the following passage from a book entitled *Counsels on Health:*

> Mothers should take their daughters into the kitchen with them when very young, and teach them the art of cooking. . . . She should instruct them patiently, lovingly, and make the work as agreeable as she can by her cheerful countenance and encouraging words of approval. . . . Their constitution will be better for such labor; their muscles will gain tone and strength, and their meditations will be more healthy and elevated at the close of the day.[29]

HOW TO EAT

In the Adventist health concept, healthful cooking is only half the equation. It is also important to know *how* to eat. And when. And even where. When people eat improperly "this calls their nervous energies to the stomach, and they have no vitality to expend in other directions."[30] They have developed a number of interesting suggestions on how to get the most benefit and enjoyment from food one eats. Not surprisingly, therefore, the first rule is *enjoy yourself.*

When eating, enjoy it. "At mealtime cast off care and anxious thought: do not feel hurried, but eat slowly and with cheerfulness, with your heart filled with gratitude."[31] What do you do if mealtime approaches and you are in a great hurry, excited, or anxious? Wait. If you eat under stress or time pressure, your overloaded system simply will not be able to handle digestion properly.[32] And for those who plead that they *never* have that kind of time, eat less, and eat slowly. Use what time you do have in eating properly rather than bolting down more food and getting less benefit from it.

They also believe that if we fail to enjoy our food, it will benefit us less. The same thing goes for worrying about one's diet, especially after a meal. Their advice? Confine your worry to the menu stage of the meal: think about getting the proper food *then,* and let dinnertime be spent free from care.

What does happiness—not just at mealtime, but in general—have to do with health? Quite a bit, according to one study. People were asked to rate how happy they generally were. At the end of nine years, 16 percent of the men who classed themselves as "not happy" were dead. The death rate was only 10.3 percent among those who thought themselves to be "very happy." The difference is a rather startling 55 percent increase in mortality—related merely to happiness. Perhaps the advice to enjoy one's-self deserves a careful second look.

By now it should be clear that this ideal concerning mealtime is far removed from fast food restaurants or from bolting food, half unaware, in front of a television screen. Mealtime is an event in which a family can join in a common, happy experience. Perhaps this is a good place to repeat that Adventists have only 42 percent as many deaths from peptic ulcers as do most Americans.

Eat slowly and thoroughly. The digestive process does, after all, begin in the mouth. A number of enzymes in the mouth are necessary for proper digestion of food, particularly starches. If this process is short circuited, the body may get less benefit.

Exercise restraint. Adventists strongly urge the need for restraint in the diet—not only in quantity but also in variety and complexity of foods. They urge that food intake be limited. Too much food does not guarantee more benefit, but it certainly does guarantee additional wear and tear on the digestive system. Adventists believe overeating to be a real health hazard—not only in causing overweight, but in more subtle ways. They teach, for example, that too much food dulls mental acuity, blunts the memory and perceptive faculties, and renders a person much less productive. Their theory is subject to rather easy verification. Think about how alert you feel after a really heavy meal.

They also urge that variety of foods be limited at each meal. They feel that three or four separate dishes are plenty of variety at one sitting, and that more than this may cause unnecessary work for the digestive system as it accommodates to the maze of chemical combinations thrust on it. For the same reason they suggest simple food, free from rich, highly seasoned dishes. (A bonus for the plan is less work for the cook.)

Avoid drinking liquids with meals. Adventists are great believers in the use of water. They employ it internally and externally, as a preventive and as a treatment for disease. But one place where they do not recommend it is at the dinner table. One reason is that when one gets in the habit of drinking with meals, the flow from the salivary glands diminishes, and enzymes necessary for proper digestion are not mixed with the food. Another reason is that liquids taken with meals are usually chilled. Studies show that chilled food passes through the stomach more rapidly, with less adequate digestion. Drinking fluids with meals can be a hard habit to break, and to aid in getting over it they recommend avoiding spicy or salty foods such as pickles and condiments. Incidentally, for these same reasons Adventists prefer firmer and drier foods to those that are more liquid. Steamed rice, for example, would be preferred over thin, watery porridge. "Taken in a liquid state, your food will not give vigor and tone to the system ..."[33] Their advice: eat more solids and less liquids.

When should one drink water? Either before or after mealtime, so as not to interfere with digestion. And drink plenty of it—six glasses a day is none too much for the average healthy individual.

Enjoy a little moderate exercise after meals. What is the very best thing to do after eating? Exercise—moderately. Find a quiet country lane, or a nice stretch of city park, and simply walk. Jogging or other demanding exercise will interfere with digestion, but a brisk walk, taken in the open air, will provide more benefits than you might imagine. For one thing, it gets your mind off your food—an important bonus for those who are inclined to worry about diet. For another, it avoids immediate heavy mental activity, which is also bad right after a meal. Neither the mind nor the body should be vigorously stressed during the early stages of digestion, because doing so draws the body's resources away from the digestive organs, where they are most needed. A walk will also burn off a few of the extra calories you may have taken in, and it will give you a chance to fill your lungs with the fresh air they seldom get in an office or shop.

Adventists who adopt this rule find it strangely addicting. Mealtime, followed by a quiet walk in natural surroundings, becomes one of the high points of the day. They say that from this break they return refreshed in mind and body, ready to put more into the work that lies ahead.

Another tip from the Adventist program: avoid eating right after heavy exertion. Digestion demands more from the system than most people realize, and heavy exercise just before a meal may prevent the digestive organs from getting the resources they need. Best, allow yourself a little time to relax before eating, and results will be better.

Space your meals by five or six hours. Adventists believe that one should never eat until the stomach has had a chance to rest from the labor of digesting the previous meal. A rule of thumb they follow is to space meals at least five or six hours apart, eating absolutely nothing between times. The period between meals is the time for water, so long as it is not drunk too soon after a meal.

At least one study bears out this concern. Over a nine-year period the death rate for men who regularly snacked between meals was 20 percent higher than for men who did not.

Try eating two meals a day. Not everyone can handle this one, but if you have a weight problem you may find that it really works in shedding pounds. Which meal do you leave out? The one taken late in the evening. Adventists frequently make breakfast the largest meal of the day, on the theory that one needs more food at the start of the work day than at the end. For many people who are used to skipping breakfast, there is a ready answer: skip supper, and breakfast will take care of itself. (A large, heavy supper is usually the reason they can't face breakfast.) If you do wish to have a third meal, make it a light one (such as fruit or bread), and be sure that it is eaten several hours before going to bed.

This point has been echoed by several prominent nutritionists and physicians. In their well-known work, *Modern Nutrition in Health and Disease,* Wohl and Goodhart say that "since his ability to assimilate his food is greater in the mornings, he should make his breakfast and his lunch the chief meals of the day."[34] A researcher in England points "an accusing finger at the evening meal as the cause of high incidence of dental cavities."[35] The Journal of the American Dietetic Association cites studies which show that workers produce more work when they have had an adequate breakfast. (Mid-morning snacks produced little or no advantage.)[36]

Special hints for office workers and Type A personalities. If your work is largely sedentary, mental, and demanding, Adventists have some special tips for you. *Don't* overeat. It is more important for you than anyone to eat sparingly, even of the best food. For you, eliminating the evening meal may be more than a health luxury—it may be a necessity. It is especially important for you to get some moderate exercise after eating; to go right from a meal to demanding mental effort will only result in blunted productivity. To put it in Adventist words, "There are men and women of excellent natural ability who do not accomplish half what they might if they would exercise self-control in the denial of appetite. . . . More than others, they need to be temperate in their eating."[37]

Eat less, exercise more, and give yourself the luxury of some time each day free from care, reserved exclusively for your own relaxation. For you, the after-dinner walk fits this description perfectly. When demands upon you are the heaviest, prescribe the strongest dietary medicine: "At each meal take only two or three kinds of simple food, and eat no more than is required to satisfy hunger. Take active exercise every day, and see if you do not receive benefit."[38]

Adventists urge eating one's heaviest meals before and during the workday, not at its end. A study shows that they are right. Groups of men and women were studied over a nine-year period. Men who rarely ate breakfast had over 40 percent greater mortality during the nine-year period than did men who usually ate a good breakfast. For women, the death rate was nearly 30 percent higher when breakfast was skipped. Adventists believe that the system is better able to handle a large quantity of food at the start of the day when food energy can be used by the body in work.

Have mealtimes at regular hours. Adventist thought is that mealtimes be held at regular hours. The body adapts very readily to natural cycles and rhythms, and seems to do best when events such as mealtime come a regular, fixed time each day. For some people this seems impossible, but it is a nice goal to try for. As long as you are setting aside a specific time, you might as well set aside enough time to make the meal the sort of relaxed, family-oriented event that they suggest.

For those who wish to change to a better eating schedule, they offer some practical advice. First, expect some discomfort for a short while. As we said, the body adapts readily to rhythms—including that of a late meal. Anticipating the arrival of food, it will probably gear up for the event, producing extra gastric juices and insulin, which will lower your blood sugar and make you feel hungry and faint. Second, fool yourself by drinking a glass or two of water, which will make the stomach feel full without adding any calories to digest. And then get busy doing something to take your mind off food. If you must think about food, think about breakfast—and *wait* for it.

Chapter 4

In Contact With Nature

Picture (if you can) an 83-year-old lady jogging at sunrise and then climbing the stairways of a nearby building while carrying a backpack filled with thirty-five pounds of rock—just before she leaves for her annual assault on California's Mt. Whitney. Try another mental picture: a surgeon who at 94 was still doing major surgery—at one of the *twenty* hospitals he built all over Asia.

You have just seen two examples of Adventist health reform at its ultimate, people who reach for nature with gusto and who, in the process, seem to have total disdain for getting old. In contact with nature: that's the title of our chapter, and that's the way they accomplish an important part of staying healthy.

SEVEN STEPS TO HEALTH

Dr. Lester Breslow, dean of the School of Health at UCLA, recently made a rather startling assertion: it is possible, with existing knowledge, to increase American life expectancy by eleven years. How? By following seven basic health principles:

1. Avoid tobacco.
2. Limit the use of alcohol.
3. Eat a good breakfast every day.
4. Avoid eating between meals.
5. Get adequate rest, from 7 to 8 hours a night.
6. Engage in frequent, regular exercise.
7. Remain close to one's ideal weight.

Researchers did a study to see whether these rules of health really correlate with life expectancy. For nine years they studied a group of men and women, comparing their life-styles with mortality rates. At the end of the nine-year period, men who regularly observed all seven rules had a death rate of only 5.2 percent. Those who followed six of the rules—only one less—had over *twice* the mortality rate. Men who observed three or fewer had a 20 percent chance of dying within the nine-year period.!

The results for women were less spectacular but still showed a direct relationship between the rules of health and life expectancy. Notice the data in table 21.

Table 21

Relation of Longevity to Health Rules

Death rate for men

Number of health rules followed	Percentage dead in 9 years
7	5.2%
6	10.6%
5	12.8%
4	14.2%
0–3	19.7%

Death rate for women

7	5.1%
6	7.2%
5	7.8%
4	10.5%
0–3	12.1%

Table 22

Exercise Pattern	Percentage Dead in 9 years	
	Men	Women
Often, vigorous	6.8%	6.5%
Often, moderate	11.8%	NA
Occasional, vigorous	12.4%	7.6%
Occasional, moderate	15.0%	8.2%
Never	18.6%	16.1%

The study also showed interesting relationships between specific health principles and longevity. For example, men who never exercised had 274 percent greater risk of death within nine years than did men who exercised often and vigorously.

Even one's pattern of rest correlates with mortality risk. Men who got eight hours of sleep a night had 40 percent less risk of death than men who got less than six hours. (Interestingly, the death rate climbs again when sleep exceeds nine hours a night, an indication, perhaps, that too much sleep may point to an underlying physiological problem—or that one can simply get too much of a good thing.)

Now compare Dr. Breslow's principles with the Adventist health program, and you find some fascinating similarities, both in context and results. Breslow suggests that by a few commonsense health habits we could give ourselves eleven extra years of life. Adventists have not achieved that goal yet, but at 6.2 extra years of male life expectancy they are further along than most. And with a few modifications, Adventist principles and Breslow's seven rules could have come from the same book. Take a look at Table 23 and the comparison will come into focus.

Table 23

Adventist Health Principles	*Breslow's "Health Habits"*
Pure air	Not smoking
Pure water	Limitation on alcohol
Careful nutrition	A good breakfast
Regularity	Limiting between-meal snacks
Rest	7–8 hours sleep
Exercise	Regular exercise
Moderation in eating	Weight control

Look over the items in table 23 and you will realize that we have already talked about a majority of them: pure water, careful nutrition, regularity in diet, and moderation in food intake—an indication of how important nutrition is, both in Dr. Breslow's thinking and in the Adventist health program. Now we'll turn to the remaining three items, exploring the ways in which Adventists meet their physical world. As we do so, we'll summarize their total life-style in table 24.

Table 24

Seventh-day Adventist Life-style

No tobacco
No alcohol
Vegetarian diet (some include milk and eggs)
No pork or pork products
Avoid:
   Caffein
   Spices and spicy foods
   Hot condiments
Emphasize:
   Whole grains, fruits, nuts, vegetables, as fresh and naturally served as
     possible

Fresh air
Exercise
Enjoyment of nature
Trust in divine power

AIR AND SUNLIGHT

Adventists believe that some of our greatest blessings (and greatest medicines) are absolutely free. At the head of the list are fresh air and sunlight.

There is nothing startling about this idea: most of us would agree with it. But do we really *use* these agencies? In most cases, probably not—at least nowhere near their capacity for usefulness. For example, how many of us make a conscious effort to breathe deeply, to sit erect so that the lungs and heart can really work, to throw open the curtains so that sunlight (which is a surprisingly powerful disinfectant) can really benefit us? In this chapter we will talk about the ways in which Adventists consciously try to use the agencies of nature, and the benefits they believe can be derived from what they do. First, the topic at hand: how do air and sunlight benefit us, and how can we use them most effectively?

Develop the habit of breathing deeply. "The strength of the system is, in a great degree, dependent upon the amount of pure, fresh air breathed. If the lungs are restricted, the quantity of oxygen received into them is also limited, the blood becomes vitiated, and disease follows."[1] Even one's posture at work affects the way in which the lungs operate; sit or stand erect, shoulders back. You may be surprised at the difference it makes in how you feel.

Open your home to air and sunlight. In an era of forced air heating and cooling, we sometimes forget that there is very limited benefit in merely recirculating the same stale, used air over and over. Adventists urge the benefits that come from open windows. They also believe that a bright, well-ventilated home will do much for both physical and mental health, especially in children.

Especially ensure a free circulation of air while you sleep. Adventists suggest that the unpleasant fatigued feeling many people have at the start of the day can be traced to sleeping in a room where there is no circulation of fresh air. They suggest that you try opening a window by small degrees until you are used to the cooler night air. Avoid a direct draft, but let the air circulate freely in the room. It may help to solve the problem of morning blahs.

Take a walk early each morning. Every morning, while the air is still cool and reasonably fresh, take a walk. Throw off the worries of the day. Reserve the time just for yourself. If you like, use some of the time for gardening, cultivating flowers or a small vegetable garden. While doing so, consciously try to breathe deeply so that you get the benefit of full respiration with your exercise. The benefits? This is "the surest safeguard against colds, coughs, congestion . . . and a hundred other diseases."[2] If all this sounds too good to be true, remember that the lungs are the organs through which much of the body's wastes and impurities are thrown off. Retain those impurities in the system through improper breathing and you are likely to have a litany of troubles. And if you do ignore these suggestions and get sick, the suggestion for recovery is the same one you ignored in the first place: "A walk, even in winter, would be more beneficial to the health than all the medicine the doctors may prescribe. . . ."[3]

Remember that the sun is your most powerful ally both in treating and preventing disease. Sunlight "is one of nature's most healing agents."[4] Adventists believe that opening one's home to daily fresh air and sunlight is an important factor in preventing disease. And while they recognize that the sick need rest and special care, they have long warned against letting sick people lie inactive and indoors for days on end. In many instances, they say, these are the very things that brought on sickness. Instead of confining the sick indoors, Adventists urge that they be gotten out into the open air. As soon as possible they should be given some light, pleasant work to do— tending a small flower bed or garden, for example—which will expose them to air and sunlight, open their pores, and get their minds off their illness. For many years they were famous for this program; their rural sanitariums, set in the midst of gardens and flowers, drew patients from all over the world. That sort of approach has a quaint aura about it now, but one cannot help wondering how much we could reduce our national health care bill if we got back to something of the sort—back to using the free agencies of nature instead of trying to avoid them through technology. Obviously there is a balance between both methods; we wonder if the balance has not swung too far in one direction.

Keep the sick room well ventilated and lighted. What we have said about air and sunlight becomes doubly important when one is sick. Failure to ventilate a sick room can delay (or prevent) recovery. *"The mind becomes despressed and gloomy, while the whole system is enervated..."* [italics supplied].[5]

Every experienced physician knows that there is a great intangible called the *will to live.* The physician authors of this book have repeatedly seen patients rally or fail, simply because that will was present or absent. The will to survive can be awesomely powerful—a terminally ill patient, for example, surviving unexplainably until a missing loved one comes to visit, after which death comes swiftly and quietly. Given that important intangible, isn't there something to be said for making the surroundings as bright and well ventilated as possible? The Adventists think so.

Their advice also extends to the quarters occupied by the aged, whose lower vitality and resistance to disease make it even more important for them to have plenty of sunlight and fresh, pure air. If the sick or aged person cannot tolerate exposure to an open window in his own room, they suggest opening a window in a room nearby so that fresh air can still circulate to benefit the person needing it.

EXERCISE

Next to diet, Adventists consider exercise the most important thing you can do to stay healthy. And their belief in exercise has produced some absolutely astonishing results. Take, for example, the Adventist doctor who at age 84 was still building hospitals, at 94 was still doing surgery, and *at 97* was perfecting improvements in soy milk, a food which he invented and which has saved the lives of thousands of infants allergic to cow's milk. His name was Harry Miller, a remarkable man who began each day with one or two hours of vigorous physical exercise. He was a colorful figure whose last full day of life was spent working in the research lab of a food manufacturer—at nearly 98 years of age!

Our second example is Hulda Crooks, an 83-year-old lady who climbs Mt. Whitney every year. Recently an NBC camera crew accompanied her to shoot some footage of this remarkable lady for the "Today Show." They encountered terrible weather—rain, hail, and snow in mid-August. They met many hikers retreating down the mountain. Near the summit, in the painful, thin air above 14,000 feet, even the cameramen had to reach for portable oxygen bottles. What was Hulda doing? Napping, nearby, on her favorite flat rock near Trail Crest. Her advice pretty well sums up the philosophy of the serious Adventist health reformer, in love with nature and with the thrill of living beyond average limits: "Be active. Get a hobby. *Do* something. Live simply and eat simply. Start when you're young and you'll be able to enjoy life when you're older."[6]

Hulda Crooks's statement sounds very similar to a passage we found in our research of Adventist writings on health—one of the most exciting passages we discovered: "If physical exercise were combined with mental exertion, the blood would be quickened in its circulation, the action of the heart would be more perfect, impure matter would be thrown off, and new life and vigor would be experienced in every part of the body."[7]

Think that statement through and profound implications emerge. Few people would deny that there is benefit in exercise. Fewer still would deny the need for mental effort. But how often do we think of those two apparently unrelated activities as impacting on each other, producing a result greater than just the sum of each?

This is a good point at which to remind ourselves that Adventists are deeply committed to the idea that the body is like a finely tuned machine, all systems of which must be stressed in just the right proportion for maximum results. Today we call this ideology "holistic health" and greet it as one of the exciting new frontiers of medicine. Adventists advanced the concept as early as the 1870s, during which the above quotation was first put into print. The body, they declare, "may be compared to nicely adjusted machinery," one part of which "should not be subjected to constant wear and pressure, while another part is rusting from inaction."[8] And then they go on to suggest that each person should measure his or her own needs most carefully, to learn just what proportion of mental effort and exercise produces best results.

Is there scientific support for the idea that the health of the nervous system is related to physical exercise? Yes. As far back as 1957, Dr. M. S. D. Michael said, in the *Journal* of the Michigan State Medical Society, that exercise should involve the *whole* body, not just specific areas, and that physical activity benefits the autonomic nervous system.[9] In the same issue of that journal, Dr. Hazen Price stated that regular and systematic exercise each day will help the individual "meet daily tasks with a better body and a more alert mind."[10]

Perhaps the most exciting statement of all comes from Dr. Henry Montage: "I think that such regular exercise would affect not only physical capacity but their interest in other people and the world around them, their energy for doing mental work and in general, their vim and vigor for carrying out everyday activity."[11]

Recall that at the start of this book we pointed out that Adventists, statistically speaking, live longer, and that they also seem to enjoy greater productivity in these extra senior years because of the benefits of good health. The medical opinions just quoted may help to explain why.

Contrast that picture of a healthy, productive old age with another picture we in the hospital industry see all too often: a patient in his 60s, helpless after a stroke, unable to recognize even his own family, and in need of expensive custodial care for the rest of his life. It is this sort of unnecessary burden that is helping to capsize our whole system of health care—a burden that can be avoided in large part by simple, commonsense rules everyone could follow.

If the Adventists are correct in assuming that the right mix of physical and mental exercise produces a multiplied effect on one's being, giving "new life and vigor" in "every part of the body," one of the greatest breakthroughs in health and productivity is right at hand, virtually cost-free, available to nearly everyone.

How does one arrange activities that use both mental and physical powers? Probably the first thought that comes to the mind of most people would be some form of mentally demanding sport—and no doubt that would serve the purpose to a point. But Adventists go a step further than this. Why not, they ask, get these benefits while engaged in some activity that produces a useful function? Listen to this statement from one of their early books on education:

> There is science in the humblest kind of work, and if all would thus regard it, they would see nobility in labor. Let the educated ability be employed in devising improved methods of work, to devise the best methods in farming, in building, and in every other department.[12]

This is pure Americana, filled with the flavor of an age in which Americans were busily inventing everything from combine harvesters to airplanes, and the words have a certain gossamer, bygone charm about them. Yet the serious Adventist also accepts them quite literally for himself. For someone who is committed to reaching an optimum level of life, it is impossible to ignore the intriguing possibility that one might exercise both mind and body, reach a more perfect state of health, and at the same time produce some lasting benefit to the world around him.

This carries over into their philosophy of training children. "Your means could not be used to better advantage than in providing a workshop furnished with tools for your boys, and equal facilities for your girls. They can be taught to love labor."[13] One way they accomplish this is in working together on family projects. Even a simple garden can provide healthful exercise while offering lessons in a whole array of fields, from botany to economics. "This real, earnest work calls for a strength of intellect as well as of muscle," they say about agriculture. "To develop the capacity of the soil requires thought and intelligence."[14]

This is an extremely broad health concept, in which one's productivity is directly related to health and happiness, and in which even common tasks offer the adventure of mind and body working together to produce something excellent. Combine exercise with mental effort. It is a rule high on their list of health priorities. It is easily stated. It is profound in effect.

Exercise the whole body. We have already seen that Adventists believe in exercising the whole body systematically—a practice borne out by recent medical research. How can this best be done?

If they had to give a single answer, safe for everyone, they would answer in one word: walking. A brisk walk, with the shoulders back and head erect, provides exercise that cannot be improved upon, in their opinion. And it is safe for nearly everyone—free from the strange litany of side effects (such as menstrual irregularity and joint difficulties) that can accompany more vigorous activities such as jogging. (Even many heart patients are discovering that walking is a simple, inexpensive form of therapy, which, combined with careful diet, can give them remarkable freedom from pain.)

Another excellent source of all-round exercise is working out of doors around a yard or garden. It offers several bonuses: fresh air and sunlight are two. A third advantage, which comes for some people as a hidden bonus, is that exercise out of doors can actually be enjoyable—and help alleviate stress. Many people equate physical fitness with dull, repetitive routines inside a stuffy gymnasium. It need not be so, and the quickest way to learn that is to try a half hour each morning in the yard or garden, working at a pace that allows one to enjoy the morning freshness while getting some useful things done.

Adventists believe that it is important not only to exercise but to *enjoy* it, and in this sense enjoyment is very much a part of exercising the whole body, muscles as well as mind. If exercise is done "without the heart's being in it . . . the benefit which should result from the exercise is not gained."[15] Their advice, therefore, would be to pick the form of activity which you most enjoy, do it with gusto, and expect good results.

We know that exercise is a strong factor in reducing the risk of heart attack. In the bloodstream there are substances known as high density lipoproteins ("HDL" for short), which are associated with lower risk of heart disease. Studies show that consistent exercise tends to raise the level of these helpful substances in the blood.

There are many other reasons for daily exercise. To illustrate the point we'll list just those that apply to the heart and vascular system. Exercise can:

Increase stroke volume, the amount of blood pumped with each heartbeat.

Decrease pulse rate, thereby giving the heart more time to rest between beats.

Increase circulation, benefiting the entire system with a greater flow of oxygen, nourishment, and removal of impurities.

Increase collateral circulation in the heart muscle, thus providing more "routes" for blood to get to the heart (and thereby reducing one's risk of heart attack).

Decrease one's risk of death in the event of heart attack.

The Greater New York Health Insurance Plan did an interesting study on the annual incidence of first-time heart attacks in men aged 35 to 64. The data is shown in table 25. Most spectacular is the fact that a smoker who exercises at least moderately seems to have less risk of heart attack than does a nonsmoker who is inactive. That is not meant as a suggestion to combine smoking with exercise; an exercising smoker still has twice the risk of an exercising nonsmoker.

Table 25

Annual Incidence of First Myocardial Infarction Age 35–64

	Least Active	Most Active
Total	8.5	4.2
Nonsmokers	6.3	3.0
Smokers	10.9	5.8
Fatality Within 48 Hours	3.8	.9

Notice especially that simply by exercising moderately, one can reduce one's risk of death in the event of heart attack by about 400 percent.

Exercise is so important that many doctors now urge their patients to engage in something called "cardiopulmonary" exercise, which can be nothing more than walking for twenty minutes' unbroken duration each day. Why walk instead of jog? Because it is an exercise safe for nearly everyone. (Some reconditioning centers have recently achieved national prominence by taking even severely ill heart patients, putting them on a strict low-fat diet, and having them walk several miles each day. At the end of a month on this regimen many of them experience relief they have not enjoyed for many years.)

The principle behind cardiopulmonary exercise is to get one's pulse rate up to a "target level" for maximum safe exercise of the heart. One way this can be determined is by a simple formula: a person's age is subtracted from the figure 200, giving a maximum pulse rate that should not be exceeded. To be extra safe, that figure is usually reduced by 10 percent. For example, if a man is 50, his age, subtracted from 200, leaves 150. An extra margin of safety is gotten by subtracting 10 percent of 150 (15), leaving a safe maximum pulse rate of 135. In exercising he should try to reach that rate, but not go above it. And to achieve meaningful benefit for the heart, he should exercise for twenty minutes without stopping. For most people that means a walk of about one mile.

And so the Adventist suggestion for a morning walk has much to commend it scientifically. It is safe for nearly everyone, it is an excellent all-round exercise, and it gives a person a stimulating start on the day when the air is still cool, invigorating, and reasonably fresh. (Unfortunately, that is a necessary consideration for the majority of our population who live in urban centers.) Morning exercise also has the great advantage that it is done first thing, before telephone calls and pressing business reduce one's exercise program to nothing but good intentions. Our suggestion is simply to *try it* every morning for a week.

If your work is sedentary, make special efforts to exercise regularly in the open air. Office workers "frequently remain too much indoors, occupying heated rooms filled with impure air. Here they employ themselves closely to study or writing, taking little physical exercise. . . . As a consequence, the blood becomes sluggish, and the powers of the mind are enfeebled. The whole system needs the invigorating influence of exercise in the open air. A few hours of manual labor each day would tend to renew the bodily vigor, and rest and relax the mind."[16] Regular, vigorous physical activity is especially recommended for students, whose intense mental application needs to be balanced with corresponding exercise.

When unable to exercise, eat sparingly. From time to time everyone is caught in circumstances that make exercise difficult or impossible. To minimize the effects of inactivity, one should try to eat less during these periods. Less food is needed, since less calories are being expended in the form of work, and excess food taken under these circumstances merely overloads the system and produces a whole list of familiar problems, including drowsiness, mental inefficiency, and greater risk of cardiovascular disease.

Try to exercise after each meal. We have already talked about this in the last chapter. Light, pleasant exercise such as a walk is of great benefit after eating. Strenuous exercise should not be taken, but a relaxing walk in the fresh air, preferably in natural surroundings, benefits digestion and refreshes the whole body.

"It will come as a shock to the sedentary male," writes Dr. Thomas Cureton, of the University of Illinois, "to learn that his body was middle aged by the time he was 26."[17] Researchers measured the circulation of blood in 500 industrial workers and discovered that by age 25, average circulation has dropped 40 percent. At age 35, the reduction is 60 percent. It would appear that Adventist concern over sedentary occupations is well founded.

Exercise even when ill. This is probably one of the more surprising bits of Adventist advice, and it needs to be explained. No one suggests heavy exercise during severe illness. But as soon as one is able, a short walk in fresh air and sunlight is their prescription for quicker recovery. Notice this interesting statement: "Physical exercise and labor combined has a happy influence upon the mind, strengthens the muscles, improves the circulation, and gives the invalid the satisfaction of knowing his own power of endurance."[18]

When people are ill, there is constant danger that they will dwell on the fact of illness until recovery may be blocked by this mental preoccupation. Many physicians freely admit that the majority of their patients have illnesses that originate largely in the mind. Adventists propose to prevent this by getting patients' minds off themselves and onto something more pleasant instead. The subject matter they choose to accomplish this mental transition is nature.

For many years Adventists were famous for their country sanitariums, set in the midst of orchards and flower gardens, where the sick were treated with simple remedies, sunlight, fresh air, and an atmosphere of quiet confidence in their recovery. At many of these sanitariums patients were given light tasks to do, such as tending a small flower bed or garden. The purpose, of course, was to give them something to occupy their time, taking their minds off their own problems. Instead of being sent to physical therapy, for ten minutes under an ultraviolet lamp (at a cost of $35), they were sent into the free sunlight and given a purpose for living. One wonders whether our present health care system, breaking under a load of $200 billion a year, might not learn some valuable lessons from those early Adventist techniques.

CIRCULATION

The importance of good circulation can hardly be overemphasized, according to the Adventists. They explain that one of the major functions of the bloodstream is to carry impurities out of the system. If the circulation is poor, waste products are not so readily expelled, nor does the body get the supply of oxygen and nourishment it needs for good health. Much of their exercise program is designed to promote healthy circulation. We'll talk now about some of the ways they try to ensure that circulation is both effective and balanced.

Use of water. For Seventh-day Adventists, water is a profound and versatile agent, used not only in prevention but also in treatment of disease. They feel that bathing accomplishes much more than just personal hygiene. It also tends to equalize circulation by drawing the blood to the surface, filling the miles of capillaries in the skin. At the same time it is drawn away from the internal organs, relieving them from congestion. The results, they believe, are freer respiration, better muscle relaxation, and a happier outlook on life. "The mind and body are alike invigorated, the intellect is made brighter, and every faculty becomes livelier."[19] Other benefits include better digestion, better resistance to colds and flu, and better general health for the internal organs because of active blood flow. If that array seems too impressive for such an ordinary thing as a bath, perhaps you haven't practiced the art the way many Adventists advise—with use of cold water as well as warm!

If a person's health is reasonably good, Adventists suggest that each bath or shower be followed by a brief shower in cold water. Here is their reasoning: during a hot bath the blood is drawn to the surface. Skin pores are opened. Circulation is stimulated, impurities are expelled. The blood is drawn away from the iternal organs. By briefly stepping into a cold shower, a person can further stimulate circulation. Blood that has accumulated at the surface now retreats to deeper tissues, the vascular system gets a second healthy workout, and the body is less subject to chill in the cold outside air. Scientists are now discovering that a cold shower has a second benefit. It temporarily results in a higher white blood cell count. Since white cells help to fight disease, that is a desirable side effect that may explain the *why* behind the Adventist statement that bathing "fortifies against colds."[20]

Adventists also employ the natural, inexpensive remedy of water when treating the sick. At one time they were world famous for their hydrotherapy techniques, employed at institutions such as the Battle Creek Sanitarium, where kings and presidents were frequent patients. There is much our modern, expensive medical care system could still learn from the early Adventist techniques of water therapy.

A liberal use of water is urged inside as well as outside the body. Good circulation will result in an enormous chemical turnover in the system. One of the main reagents the body uses is water, both as a chemical and as a vehicle for getting other chemicals where they need to go, and the body needs a surprisingly large supply, from 4 to 6 glasses a day. However, do not have your main intake of water at mealtimes, when it will dilute digestive enzymes and slow the absorption of food. Water—and plenty of it—is taken between meals as a handy way for compulsive snackers to feel full without adding calories.

Dress carefully. Interestingly, Adventists also feel that a person's mode of dress has much to do with healthy circulation. If the extremities are overly exposed, particularly in cold weather, the capillaries constrict in an effort to conserve body warmth. The heart, forced to pump blood through these narrowed vessels, has to work harder. As the blood passes through exposed surfaces, it loses heat and draws on the body's reserves to regain normal temperature. The process repeats itself until the system falls behind in the cooling-heating-cooling cycle. The results are habitually cold hands, legs, and feet—and a habitual liability to colds and flu. What advice is offered on dress? "If any part of the body should be favored with extra coverings, it should be the limbs and feet."[21] They believe that habitually chilled feet and legs result in circulatory imbalances and a greater likelihood of disease.

Get plenty of fresh air. The old standby, morning exercise in fresh air, applies to circulation as well as to other areas of health. Brisk exercise such as walking stimulates rapid circulation in the entire body. Imagine a day begun with a hot and cold shower, after a good night's sleep, an appetite allowed to bloom by eliminating a late, heavy meal the night before, a brisk walk in the fresh air just before breakfast—and you have captured the typical morning of an Adventist health reformer. They believe that this helps their outlook for the whole day.

"Brisk, yet not violent, exercise in the open air, with cheerfulness of spirits, will promote the circulation, giving a healthy glow to the skin, and sending the blood, vitalized by the pure air, to the extremities."[22]

Avoid overeating. It should be obvious, but judging from the typical American profile, it is not: overweight does disastrous things to circulation. First, there is more apt to be excess fat in the blood, making it thick, sticky, and slow to circulate. Secondly, each pound of excess fat adds incredible numbers of blood vessels and capillaries, all of which have to serviced by the overworked heart. Excess food is probably one of our greatest health hazards in America today, and it is the one most immediately within everyone's control. Adventists warn that "your health is greatly injured by overeating and eating at improper times,"[23] and they characteristically link the effects to the mind: "overeating produces circulatory imbalances which affect mental acuity." One wonders if we will ever count up all the health advantages to be gained from simple moderation in our intake of food.

STIMULANTS AND DRUGS

Stimulants. Under that category come a proliferating host of substances, many of which are in common use today. Some are mild—the morning cup of coffee, for example, to which people have become so accustomed that the effects of a single cup may be barely noticeable. Others are potent, very new, and filled with medical uncertainties. All are avoided by Adventists. Their reasons for doing so are interesting.

At first sight, the topic of stimulants seems more related to diet than to a chapter on fresh air, exercise, and perceptions of nature. But think it through: few stimulants are taken as food. They are basically used to produce an effect on one of two things: how we feel, or how we perceive reality. By now you should have concluded that one of the Adventists' major preoccupations is reality—discovering it, enjoying it, working with it. Altering one's perception of reality through any stimulant is, therefore, a bit of intellectual dishonesty most Adventists cannot bring themselves to commit.

If that sounds extreme, remember that this is a group of people who believe that life's best gifts come from the closest possible adherence to natural law. They are, therefore, uniquely dependent on truth—and therefore on an accurate perception of it. In a sense they carry a little bit of everyone with them in that philosophy. Few people would argue, for example, that one is less safe driving a car after four martinis than when cold sober. Why? Because a chemical has intervened to affect the driver's perception of reality. Adventists take that to its logical conclusion, and ask a question that is difficult to answer: if such chemicals can affect my safety during a purely mechanical act such as driving, won't they also endanger my capacity to make more demanding moral or intellectual judgments? One can always raise the argument of moderation. But moderation is a terribly subjective thing, colorable by a person's wishes, moods, or ungovernable drives such as alcoholism. Adventists solve the problem instantly and conclusively: they avoid it totally in the first place.

In this section we will discuss stimulants as they see them: what they are (some surprises); what they do in the system; and how to do without them. We will include some items not always thought of as stimulants *per se*.

Tobacco. In 1864, when tobacco was frequently taken as a medication for the lungs, Seventh-day Adventists were warned that "Tobacco is a poison of the most deceitful and malignant kind, all the more dangerous because its effects upon the system are so slow, and at first scarcely perceivable."[24] In 1905 they were again warned that "Tobacco is a slow, insidious, *but most malignant poison*" [italics supplied].[25] Notice that in both instances the word *malignant* is conspicuously present—a caution given nearly 100 years before the surgeon general's warning that cigarettes and lung cancer are statistically linked. Today we know even more than was known when that warning was first issued. Cancer of the bladder also seems to be related to smoking, as does oral cancer, laryngeal cancer and esophageal cancer. Some new evidence suggests that smoking may also be linked with pancreatic cancer—a terrible, virulent form of the disease with a five-year survival rate of only 1 percent. (This one has officials worried: pancreatic cancer has increased recently by 20 percent and is now the fifth worst cancer killer among men.)

By far the worst killer, however, is lung cancer. Over the past forty-five years the death rate for men has shot up twenty-five times. It is now increasing dramatically for women. Survival prospects are dismal, only 8 percent for men, 12 percent for women. To put it in blunt terms, if you come down with the disease, your odds of living out five years are stacked *ten-to-one* against you.

Nor are the effects felt only by the tobacco user. Adventists have long expressed concern for children whose parents use tobacco and who are thus subjected to large amounts of sidestream smoke from their parents' cigarettes, as well as to prenatal doses of nicotine from the mother's bloodstream. In an early booklet they warned that tobacco acts on some children "as a slow poison, and affects the brain, heart, liver, and lungs." As a result some will develop chronic illness and debility. Others, they declare, will suffer sudden death.

Such cautions might be dismissed as extreme when found in a document over 100 years old. But note this statement by the American Cancer Society, issued in 1978: "Smoking by pregnant women is particularly hazardous for their unborn children. Nicotine and carbon monoxide from cigarettes can retard fetal growth, and lower-than-normal birth weight can affect a child's physical and emotional development. Women who smoke during pregnancy also increase the chances of having a stillborn infant, or a baby who dies soon after birth."[26]

Finally, Adventists deplore tobacco because it has effects that are broader, in their opinion, than just the risk of cancer. They believe that it also affects the nervous system. "It excites and then paralyzes the nerves. It weakens and clouds the brain. Often it affects the nerves in a more powerful manner than does intoxicating drink. It is more subtle, and its effects are difficult to eradicate from the system."[27] Our hospital runs a continuing program designed to help people stop smoking. After watching hundreds of them struggle with the habit, we find that statement hard to dispute.

And now research is conclusively linking tobacco and heart disease. Dr. Carl Becker of the New York Hospital-Cornell Medical Center has recently reported a study showing that a substance in tobacco reacts within the system to make blood vessel walls more permeable. This may contribute to atherosclerosis. The body's reaction to cigarette smoke can also produce irregular heart rhythms, lower blood flow to the heart muscle, and hardening of the arteries. These are the raw materials for America's number one killer—heart attack. They are aggravated by carbon monoxide in smoke lessening the amount of oxygen received by the heart.

Because its effects are so profound, so dangerous, and so broadly systemic, Adventists condemn the use of tobacco in any form. Most of their health principles are permissive; church members can adopt them or not, as they choose. This one is not. To be a member in good standing one cannot use tobacco at all.

Tea and Coffee. Recently the Food and Drug Administration issued a startling statement: they are actively considering a new regulation that would require a warning label on tea and coffee. The hazard? Birth defects.

A number of tests have now been completed that link caffeine with such birth deformities as missing fingers, cleft palate, even heart defects. The studies, conducted on both animals and humans, suggest that five cups a day could have "significant" effects on an unborn child. Each year several hundred thousand pregnant women probably drink that much and more. The implications have at least some scientists worried.

That is one example out of many supporting an early Adventist stand against the use of tea, coffee, and caffeine in other forms such as cola drinks. (Interestingly, the FDA is not considering banning caffeine from colas—one way of cutting down on consumption of the drug.) Let us give you a sampling of Adventist thinking on caffeine.

"Tea and coffee do not nourish the system. The relief obtained from them is sudden, before the stomach has time to digest them." The result? "Increased action to the heart, and short-lived energy to the entire system. All this is false strength, that we are the worse for having."[28] You might say that they consider the use of such stimulants as borrowing from future strength, a sort of deficit financing by which we are continually borrowing, never catching up, and finally suffering the result in lost health. Their alternative is simple and natural: eat less in the evening, get a good night's rest, start the day with exercise and the stimulation of a cold shower, and look forward to your work with enthusiasm. They guarantee better results, with no mortgage against tomorrow's strength.

Because stimulants temporarily produce some apparently beneficial results, many people conclude that they really need them, and continue their use. But Adventists believe that there is always a reaction. The nervous system, having been unduly excited, borrows power for present use from its future resources. All this temporary invigoration of the system is followed by a corresponding depression. It is also followed, in many instances, by headache, wakefulness, palpitation of the heart, indigestion, trembling of the nerves, and other complaints doctors hear about every day.

Another effect, of which they warn, is the action of caffeine on the brain. Their writings frequently refer to temporary exhilaration followed by a corresponding depression as the effects of caffeine wear off. They feel that the effect of all these ups and downs is a state where "the mind becomes enervated . . . the activity of the brain is greatly lessened."[29] They also avoid caffeine because it can be a hard habit to break, and they resent any agent that lessens people's control over their own will.

Their next objection to caffeine may come as a surprise. Many Adventists feel that a rich diet, high in meat, heavily spiced, and washed down with coffee or tea leads one to be more apt to use tobacco and alcohol. A few years ago some research scientists decided to see if experimentation could disclose even a particle of truth in that statement. A diet of hamburgers, hot dogs, sugar, ice cream and salty junk foods were mixed in a food blender, dried, made into powdered food, and fed to laboratory rats. Into each cage went two drinking tubes, one filled with water, the other with alcohol. After a few days on their special diets, the rats began consuming alcohol in preference to water. Then the researchers added coffee and spices. Within days alcohol consumption had shot up to the level of pure alcoholism.

Careful scientists do not offer one animal study as proof of human physiological reactions. But some mechanism is obviously at work here, and many scientists are concerned about it. Even Pavlov, the famous Russian psychologist, once called coffee "bad habit glue."

Today new evidence on the dangers of caffeine continues to accumulate. Just recently a medical journal reported the findings of a physician in Ohio. For female patients with fibrocystic breast disease, he prescribed a diet completely free from foods containing caffeine and associated drugs. Within six months, 65 percent of these patients showed complete recovery from symptoms—confirmed by physical examination, mammography, and ultrasound echograms.[30] Other researchers feel that there is a link between coffee and bladder cancer. Still others think it may be linked to colon cancer because of chemical reactions it sets up in the bowel.

And so the evidence continues to build, substantiating the Adventist position. Their ideas may anger some, particularly powerful industries that make billions of dollars a year from our American dietary habits, but they do not let this bother them unduly. They even have a reply for the person who, on his 100th birthday, attributes long life to coffee, cigars and rye whiskey: those who use unhealthful stimulants "may sometimes live to an old age, but this fact is no argument in favor of the use of these stimulants." Why? Because of "what these persons might have accomplished, but failed to do because of their intemperate habits."[31]

Alcohol and drugs. Another absolute taboo among Adventists is alcohol. One cannot be a church member in good standing while using it. First, it poses a number of health hazards, such as cirrhosis of the liver, esophageal cancer, and dependent alcoholism. Secondly, it profoundly affects one's mind, perception, and judgment.

Among the more recently discovered health hazards posed by alcohol is heart trouble. Physicians are now studying a disorder they call the "holiday heart syndrome," a distressing condition that can progress into full-scale impairment of the heart muscle. Each year around the holidays, alcohol consumption goes up. Many people, otherwise moderate in their drinking habits, use alcohol heavily at that time. Soon thereafter they begin to notice annoying irregularities in heart rhythm. Often the symptoms are so acute that they seek medical help. With abstinence the symptoms usually disappear, only to show up again at the next big indulgence. After several weeks of heavy drinking, signs of impaired contraction of the heart muscle begin to develop.[32] Adventists believe that the hazards go even further than this, and that when alcohol is used, "the system is not able to resist disease in its original God-given power.[33]

As with tobacco, their concern extends not only to the alcohol user but to the children as well. They especially warn about the hazards of drinking during pregnancy. They advance the interesting theory that this predisposes the unborn child to the use of alcohol, a legacy that can create almost insurmountable problems for the child in later life.

Is there any truth to this? Researchers probed the theory a bit with a study on laboratory rats. One group was given normal food and water; the other got increasing doses of alcohol. After a time rats from each group were mated. The offspring from the group whose parents had gotten water were given a choice between water and alcohol; they showed little interest in the alcohol. Offered the same choice, the offspring from the second group routinely chose alcohol over water. (Interestingly, this effect persisted even after the "alcoholic" parents were taken entirely off alcohol—a worrisome hint of permanent genetic change.)

Adventists believe that something similar happens with human beings, and that parents must therefore be extremely careful with their own lives because more than their own welfare is at stake. "Parents may have transmitted to their children tendencies which will make more difficult the work of educating and training these children to be strictly temperate," they advise, and if that is the case, then an even greater responsibility rests upon them to counteract earlier mistakes.[34]

And now scientists are worried that similar effects may come from the use of marijuana and other drugs. In July 1978, an international symposium at Reims, France, heard researchers from fourteen countries express concern that marijuana may have injurious effects on cellular metabolism and brain functions. Scientists are also studying the possibility that these drugs may cause genetic damage, resulting in abnormal offspring. Monkey studies show that marijuana is associated with a significant increase in dead or dying offspring, as well as genetically damaged surviving offspring.[35] The worrisome question is whether the same mechanisms will prove to operate in human beings.

For these reasons, Adventists avoid illicit drugs as totally as they avoid alcohol.

Meat: The inclusion of meat in a discussion of stimulants is bound to surprise you. First, be well aware that Adventists do not classify meat in the same objectionable category as tobacco and alcohol. They do not make the use of meat an issue in church membership, as they do in the other two instances. But they do consider it a stimulant, and so we'll talk about it from that point of view.

We probably give animals credit for far less intelligence than they actually have. Consider the conditions under which most animals are slaughtered for meat. They are taken from the natural surroundings to which their instincts have adapted them and put into crowded feedlots where the only realities are food, excreta, a terrible stench, and the crush of thousands of others like them, also in this strange predicament. From there they are prodded into trucks or railcars for what must be a terrifying journey that culminates at a slaughterhouse, heavy with the smell of death. There may be some who don't know what is coming, but probably very few.

The most basic instinct in any living thing is survival, a motive that marshals all of the awesome powers of life. Heart rate shoots up. So does respiration. The whole vascular system constricts. The adrenal glands gush hormones into the system, enabling it to accomplish feats far in excess of normal capacity. Adrenalin is a powerful drug. It is used by physicians in treating cases of severe shock. And when meat animals are at their worst, with this powerful chemical spread throughout their entire system, they are slaughtered. It pervades every bit of tissue, and it is taken in with the meat people eat.

With that scenario in mind, take a look at the Adventist view of meat as a stimulant: "Tea, coffee, and flesh meats produce an immediate effect . . . the nervous system is excited, and, in some cases, for the time being, the intellect seems to be invigorated and the imagination to be more vivid."[36]

People sometimes find it difficult to cease eating meat. They will exhibit symptoms of withdrawal for a time, as their systems acclimate to a less stimulating diet. Adventists recognize this, and even though they urge a meat-free diet for best health, they also advise people to make the change in an orderly and systematic way, substituting the very best foods available while they readjust.

OUTDOOR LIFE

As you may have surmised, most Adventists are deeply in love with nature, partly because of its beauty, partly because they see behind it an intelligence they admire, and partly because it is their form of recreation, an alternative to the more artificial forms of entertainment they usually avoid. On Saturdays, when they have free time to be together, you will often see them walking with their children, enjoying the quiet of a park or the color of changing seasons. It is a life they relish, their reward for the week's work.

Their relationship with nature is profound, and it is only partially understandable unless you see within it their belief in a loving, creative Mind from which it draws its order and its power. Their love for nature leads them to idealize a country life. Not all can arrange that ideal, but many do. They believe that man is not designed to be "crowded into cities, huddled together in terraces and tenements,"[37] and they try hard to locate in a country atmosphere, particularly if they have children.

One of the advantages they see in country living is the opportunity to grow at least some of one's own food—not merely for the pleasure of eating truly fresh garden produce, but for the lessons it offers to young and old alike. To watch a garden develop, to care for it, to be responsible, and at last to use it in sustaining your own life, is a process that leaves indelible impressions on the mind. For a child, they feel that there is no better practical training, no better way to illustrate what awaits them in life.

There is an added bonus, of course: the food from your own garden is both free from chemical hazards and delightfully fresh.

Contact with nature is a concept that can have far-reaching implications.

Epilogue

It is evening. Beneath my office window the lights of the city come on gently, broken by the lace of tule fog that haunts our valley every winter. It has been many months since I decided that a book needed to be written about health—long months, filled with challenges both in health care and in the larger arena of world events. Things are changing, faster than I thought they would.

I recall that morning, last May, when I turned off my office light to watch the sunrise. I do the same thing again—only now I see sunset, morose through the winter fog. The window goes dark, emptiness spangled with blurry lights. I think of the book we have just written. And I think of you. Perhaps you know an Adventist. You may even know some who do not follow the principles we have uncovered in our research. If so, that's too bad; you deserve a better view of a truly fascinating concept of health.

And I think about the programs our hospital has been conducting for people in our small city. For many months we've been holding free and low-cost public programs designed to minimize risk of heart attack and other diseases. We've shown people how to exercise and how to eat more healthfully. We've been putting into practice many of the principles this book describes, just to see if we *can* make a difference, if people *can* be given the gift of extra years and a more productive life. And we have come to a happy conclusion: the program works; everything we've described is possible.

Today in the early hours of morning, when the air is fresh and the day is filled with an atmosphere of new beginning, we can see people all over our city walking—with the unmistakable, purposeful attitude of people determined to change their lives for the better. Bakeries in town have told us they have a hard time keeping a stock of whole grain breads. Sale of items such as tofu is way up. (One night, recently, when we were going to put on a cooking demonstration for the public, *we* couldn't find any tofu to buy; the stores were all sold out.) But the real reward comes when people in their sixties return to our programs exclaiming that they have never felt better in their lives. That happens often—and it makes all the effort worthwhile. We are committed to health education. We have seen it work.

Sunset. The day has ended. But for us, in Bakersfield, it is really only a beginning. Because here, thousands of people have already learned that they, too, can have six extra years.

That is the best gift we can offer our community.

APPENDIX

Menu Guidelines

Breakfast

1. Oatmeal waffles
   Fruit topping
   Little Links or Stripples★
   O.J. or skim milk
   Pero or Caphag

2. Scrambled Tofu
   Stripples★
   Whole wheat toast with corn oil margarine
   Hash brown potatoes (bake in oiled waffle iron)
   O.J.
   Pero or Caphag
   Fresh Peaches

3. "Creamed Beef" on Whole Wheat Toast or Brown Rice
   Mixed nuts (dry roasted)
   Tomato juice
   ½ cantaloupe filled with fresh strawberries
   Pero or Caphag
   Whole Wheat Crunchies

★Vegetable protein meat substitutes available in health food stores or supermarket dietary sections.

Dinner

1. Tamale pie
   Tossed salad
   Deluxe Pinto Beans
   Spanish Rice
   Skim milk (optional)

2. Stuffed Green Peppers with Tomato Sauce or Ala Pilaf
   Baked yams
   Peas
   Whole wheat rolls with corn oil margarine
   Black olives, sliced tomatoes sprinkled with onion salt and dill
   weed, carrot sticks, celery sticks, radish flowers.

3. Savory Steaks or Mofidrah
   Baked potatoes with Soyonnaise
   Stuffed Tomato Salad or sliced tomatoes
   Tossed salad
   String beans with slivered almonds
   Whole wheat rolls with sesame seeds and corn oil margarine

BREAKFAST IDEAS

Granola

2 cups dates (chopped in ¾ cup water)
¾ cup corn oil
1 tablespoon liquid lecithin
1 cup sunflower seeds
1 cup wheat germ
½ cup soy flour
½ cup corn meal
½ cup sesame seeds
¼ cup flax seed
1 cup slivered almonds
½ cup chopped brazil nuts
1 teaspoon salt
1 tablespoon vanilla
8 cups oatmeal

Heat chopped dates until soft and blend in blender. Remove and mix blended dates with oil and lecithin. (Do not put oil and lecithin in blender.) Mix with dry ingredients. Bake at 250° for ½ hour, 200 for 1½ hours. Leave oven door open slightly (slip knife in door). Flavor can be improved by letting mixture stand overnight before baking or can be frozen and baked later. Add some raisins after baking, if desired. Eat with skim milk like dry cereal.

Fruit Gold

12 ounces dried apricots
12 ounces dried prunes (pitted)
5 tablespoons tapioca (heaping)
3 cups unsweetened fruit juice (pineapple and apple, or just one)
1 small can crushed pineapple

Soak apricots and prunes overnight in just enough water to cover fruit. Cook fruit slowly for one hour. Add tapioca and let cook. Remove from heat and add fruit juice and pineapple. Serve over whole wheat toast, granola, or brown rice. Slice some bananas on top. Leftovers can be frozen.

Fruit Soup

1 46-ounce can pineapple juice and juice (light syrup variety) from
fruit listed below
¾ cup minute tapioca
1 #2½ can sliced peaches
1 #2½ can sliced apricots
1 #2½ can sliced pears
1 #2½ can sliced crushed pineapple
1 #2½ can sliced fruit cocktail (optional)

Slowly bring juice and tapioca to a boil, stirring to prevent burning.
Remove from heat as soon as it comes to a full boil. Stir in fruit that
has been cut into bite-size pieces. Serve warm or cold, plain, or with
sliced bananas over granola, whole wheat toast, or brown rice.

Toasty Oats

1 cup water
⅓ cup corn oil
1 teaspoon salt
4 cups quick oatmeal

Emulsify water and oil by beating with a fork. Add dry ingredients
and mix well. Roll to ¼" thick on floured board with floured rolling
pin. (Knead lightly before rolling if too sticky.) Cut with cookie
cutter and bake at 350° until light brown—about 15 minutes. Serve
hot or cold. Good for school lunches.

Nut Milk

¼-⅓ cup nuts (blanched almonds, walnuts, or cashews)
2 cups Water
Pinch of salt
2-3 dates
1 banana for flavor (optional)

Blend above ingredients in blender. This is nice over cereal.

Scrambled Tofu

1 19-ounce package Tofu
1 tablespoon Home Style Chicken Seasoning (page 103)
1 tablespoon olive oil

Drain tofu 15-20 minutes. Crumble by squeezing through fingers into a skillet with 1 tablespoon olive oil and add seasoning. Scramble like eggs and cook until desired degree of moisture and texture are obtained. (Longer cooking makes it more dry and chewy).

Serve plain like scrambled eggs or add any one or combinations of the following ingredients:

Fresh tomato wedges—add just before serving
Fresh sliced mushrooms or 1 4-ounce can mushrooms
Fresh parsley
Fresh sliced green onion
Fresh sliced bell pepper
Baco bits
Sliced olives

This can be used in place of scrambled eggs in every recipe (i.e., fried rice, etc.)

Chicken-Garbanzo Gravy Sauce

¾ cup whole wheat flour
¼ cup olive or corn oil
2 tablespoons Savorex
1 teaspoon onion salt
1 quart broth (juice from garbanzos and mushrooms plus water to equal 1 quart)
2 cups diced frozen or canned chicken style Soyameat
1 13-ounce can garbanzos

Brown flour in large sauce pan and add oil. Stir in seasonings and broth. Add chicken, garbanzos, and mushrooms. Serve over brown rice or whole wheat toast. Serve this with fruit in season for a long-lasting breakfast.

Oatmeal Waffles

2 cups water
2 tablespoons Soyagen (heaping)
2 tablespoons oil
½ teaspoon salt
2 cups old-fashioned oats

Blend above ingredients in blender. Cook in waffle iron for 10 minutes. Waffle iron should be well oiled with Crisco or Pam the first time it is used to make these waffles. Do not raise lid before 10 minutes.

Toppings
Fresh peaches and bananas
Peanut butter and hot or cold applesauce
Apricot-date jam
Frozen orange juice diluted with half the amount of water suggested on can, thickened with cornstarch. Dice in fresh orange and serve as hot syrup.
Unsweetened grape-pear juice thickened with corn starch; add fresh or frozen blueberries or other berries and serve as hot syrup.
Fresh persimmons
Fresh fruit in season. Mash some to make juicy.

Creamed "Beef" on Whole Wheat Toast

4 ounces smoked beef—like frozen Soyameat
3 tablespoons corn oil
3 tablespoons whole wheat flour
2-2½ cups nonfat or soy milk
⅛ teaspoon Bakon yeast
⅛ teaspoon salt

Cut or tear Soyameat into small pieces. Sauté in oil (may omit) until lightly browned. Add flour and mix well. Add milk gradually, stirring constantly. Add seasonings and cook while stirring over medium heat until thickened. Serve over toast cups, toast, waffles, or brown rice.

Whole Wheat Crunchies

5½ cups water
5 tablespoons liquid lecithin
2 cups corn oil
12 cups quick oats
12 cups whole wheat flour
2 teaspoons salt

Combine oil, lecithin and water in bowl with fork. (Do not put in blender.) Combine dry ingredients and then add liquid. Roll on bottom of large baking pan to about ¼" thick (thinner if desired). Cut in squares and sprinkle lightly with salt, if desired. Bake at 300° F. for about 30 minutes. Watch closely. Good for school lunches.

Date Muffins

1 yeast cake
1 cup hot water
¼ cup corn oil
1 cup quick oats
½ teaspoon salt
1¾ cup whole wheat flour
1 cup chopped dates

Dissolve yeast in ¼ cup warm water. Mix all ingredients and beat until smooth. Put into oiled muffin tins until half full. Let rise until double. Bake at 350° F. for 20 minutes. Good for sack lunches.

Whole Wheat

Cook in pressure cooker or put in thermos bottle with boiling water the night before. Serve with nut milk and chopped dates.

DINNER SUGGESTIONS

Savory Steaks

1 19-ounce can vegetable protein steaks (many brands available)
1 onion, chopped
1 4-ounce can mushrooms, stems and pieces, or fresh
½ cup whole wheat flour
¼ cup Torumel yeast
2-3 cups water
1 tablespoon Savorex
½ cup Soyannaise (see page 102)

Place steaks in flat baking dish as they come from the can. Sauté onions and mushrooms in corn oil. Add whole wheat flour and yeast to mushrooms and onions. Mix well. Add water to make gravy. Add Savorex and Soyannaise. Pour over steaks and bake at 350° F. for ½ hour.

Steaks may be cut into strips and put into gravy to make stroganoff. Serve over brown rice, whole wheat noodles, patty shells, or toast.

Deluxe Pinto Beans

3 cups pinto beans
6 cups water
1 medium onion, chopped
1 tablespoon chopped bell pepper
2 cups tomatoes or tomato puree
1 ½ teaspoon salt
½ teaspoon each oregano, sweet basil, and cumin
1 bay leaf
1 clove garlic (optional)

Pick beans and wash in sieve. Place in 4-5-quart kettle and add 6 cups hot water. Let stand at least two hours, drain, and add enough hot water to cover beans. Add remaining ingredients; bring to a boil. Turn heat to lowest setting and cook 2 hours or until well done. May add meat extender or Vegeburger for chili style.

Stuffed Green Peppers

½ onion, chopped
2 stalks celery, diced
¼ cup diced green pepper
2 teaspoons corn oil
½ quart tomatoes
¼ cup tomato puree (or more)
¼ teaspoon each oregano and basil
1 teaspoon each Savorex, Torumel yeast, honey, and salt
Dash of thyme, marjoram, and sage
¼ cup Vegeburger (optional)
3 cups cooked brown rice
6 medium green peppers

Saute onion, celery, and diced green pepper in corn oil. Add tomatoes and tomato puree. Simmer. Add seasonings. Stir in Vegeburger, if desired. Mix this mixture with rice. Parboil whole green
peppers for 8 minutes. Remove from heat. Stuff whole or half
peppers, as desired. Bake in 9 x 12 baking dish filled with ¼ inch
water at 350° F. for 30 minutes. Serve with Tomato Sauce.

Tomato Sauce

1 6-ounce can tomato paste
¼ teaspoon sweet basil
⅛ teaspoon oregano
⅛ teaspoon dill weed
½ teaspoon salt

Simmer 10-15 minutes over low heat and serve hot over peppers.

Ala Pilaf

1 cup chopped celery
8 green onions, thinly sliced
¼ cup corn oil
2 cups ala bulgur wheat
2 cups vegetable broth or bouillon
(1 teaspoon Savorex/1 cup hot water)
1 cup slivered almonds
1 teaspoon salt
¼ teaspoon marjoram
½ teaspoon oregano
2 cups boiling water

Brown celery and onions lightly in corn oil. Add ala bulgur wheat
and brown. Add bouillon and simmer until wheat is nearly done and
flaky. Blend in almonds, seasonings and remaining water. Cover in
baking dish and bake at 325° for 1½ hours.

Tamale Pie

1 #2½ can solid pack tomatoes and juice
1 #2 can yellow whole kernel corn and juice
½ cup olive or corn oil
1 ⅔ cup yellow cornmeal
1½ cup water (may use olive juice as part of water, if desired)
1 cup Soyagen powder
1 large onion
1 teaspoon salt
1 can whole pitted black olives
1 can Vegeburger (optional)

Cook tomatoes, corn, oil and cornmeal until mixture thickens. In
blender, mix water, powder, onion, and salt. Add to the first mixture and mix well, then add olives. May add Vegeburger if desired.
Bake in oiled casserle for 1 hour at 350°. Freeze before baking if you
don't need the entire recipe.

Stuffed Tomato Salad

2½ pounds frozen soyameat chicken, medium ground or finely diced
1 cup diced celery
½ cup Soyannaise (more if needed)
½ teaspoon salt
1 tablespoon chopped green onion
1 tablespoon lemon juice
¼ teaspoon dill weed

Mix above ingredients. Core 20 small tomatoes. Cut halfway down into four sections to make tomato flower. Fill with stuffing and garnish with olive ring, parsley, paprika, etc. May also serve a scoop of stuffing on a thick tomato slice.

Soyannaise

1 cup water
½ cup Soyagen powder
½ teaspoon salt
⅓ cup corn oil
2-3 tablespoons lemon juice

Blend water, powder, and salt in blender. *Slowly* add corn oil and *rapidly* add lemon juice.

Mojedrah

2 cups dry brown rice
1 cup dry lentils
1 large onion, chopped and sautéed in olive oil
6 cups water
2 teaspoons salt
2 tablespoons Brewer's yeast

Cook rice and lentils at rolling boil for 5-10 minutes. Add sautéed onions, salt, and yeast. Cover and cook over low heat for 1 hour.

Put leftovers in casserole and heat at 350° F. for ½ hour.

Wheat and Rice Armenian

1 medium onion, chopped
½ pound soyameat chicken (Loma Linda or Worthington), diced
1 8-ounce can mushrooms
2 cups cooked long grain brown rice
1 cup wild rice (optional)
2 cups cooked whole wheat
½ cup whole wheat flour
2 tablespoons corn oil
3 cups hot water
1 tablespoon Savorex
1 ½ tablespoon Home-style Chicken Seasoning

Simmer onions in corn oil. Add diced chicken and simmer until slightly browned. Add sliced mushrooms, rice, and wheat. Simmer on low heat for 30 minutes.

Brown flour in sauce pan and add corn oil. Add water. Simmer until mixture begins to thicken. Add Savorex and Home Style Chicken Seasoning. Pour sauce into wheat and rice mixture. Place in large casserole and garnish with large mushrooms. Bake at 350°F.for 30 minutes. Yield: 20 servings.

Home Style Chicken Seasoning

¼ cup each celery salt, onion powder, and parsley flakes
1 tablespoon Tumeric
½ cup salt
1 teaspoon each garlic powder, marjoram, savory

Mix contents in 20-ounce jar and store in spice cupboard, tightly sealed.

Spanish Rice

½ cup shredded green bell pepper
½ cup chopped onions
2 tablespoons olive oil
1 cup pimento, cut in strips
½ teaspoon salt
¼ cup sliced green pitted olives
2 cups cooked brown rice
1 ½ cups canned tomatoes
Lemon slices

Mix all ingredients well. Bake in oiled baking dish with lemon slices on top at 375° F. for 30 minutes.

Italian Stuffed Mushrooms

2 pounds large whole fresh mushrooms
1 tablespoon olive oil
½ teaspoon Italian seasoning
½ small onion, diced
2 tablespoons chopped parsley
⅛ teaspoon oregano
Sprinkle of garlic salt
2 teaspoons onion salt
½ cup fine, dry bread crumbs (optional)

Clean mushrooms, remove stems, and dice stems finely. Sauté in olive oil with onions. Add remaining ingredients. Add 1-2 tablespoons lemon water to moisten if bread crumbs used. Brush mushroom caps with melted margarine and salt with onion salt. Bake in oiled baking dish at 400° for 15 minutes.

Salad Dressings

French Dressing, Cooked

Stir into 2 cups water in saucepan:

2 tablespoons cornstarch
1 tablespoon salt
4½ teaspoons paprika
½ cup lemon juice
¼ cup salad oil

Stir frequently until boiling and slightly thickened. Shake well before using.

Yield: Approximately 2½ cups. Calories: 15 per tablespoon.

Tomato Dressing

Heat to boiling:

½ cup tomato juice
1 tablespoon cornstarch

Add and cook until thick:

1 tablspoon lemon juice
1 teaspoon sugar
½ teaspoon celery salt
1 tablespoon corn oil
¼ teaspoon salt

Yield: ¾ cup

Calories: 14 per tablespoon

French Dressing, Uncooked

Combine in glass jar:

¾ cup corn oil
1 teaspoon sugar
½ teaspoon paprika
⅓ cup lemon juice
1 teaspoon salt

Shake well until blended. Chill and shake well before serving.

Yield: 1 cup.

Tomato French Dressing

½ cup tomato puree
½ cup oil (¼ cup olive oil, ¼ cup corn oil, 1 tablespoon sesame oil)
¼ cup lemon juice
1 teaspoon onion powder
½ teaspoon salt
1 tablespoon honey
½ teaspoon garlic powder

Mix well and chill.

Zero Salad Dressing

Combine in jar with tight lid:

½ cup tomato juice
½ teaspoon Accent
1 teaspoon each dehydrated onion, parsley
2 tablespoons lemon juice
1 teaspoon food yeast
Salt to taste

Yield: ⅔ cup

Creamy Italian Dressing

Fill salad dressing cruet with fresh squeezed lemon juice in place of water and vinegar. Add corn oil to a little below oil line. Add 1 teaspoon salt and favorite herbs. Shake well and serve.

For the Sweet Tooth

Date Bars

½ cup date sugar
1¼ cup quick oats, or old-fashioned oats
1 cup whole wheat flour
½ teaspoon salt
½ cup corn oil
1 cup hot water
2 tablespoons lemon juice
½ cup chopped walnuts or pecans
1 pound dates, finely ground

Combine the date sugar, oats, whole wheat flour, salt and oil for dry mixture.

For date butter filling, mix water and lemon juice with ground dates in saucepan and simmer until smooth.

Using a 9 x 11 baking dish, press half of dry mixture into dish to even depth. Spread warm date butter over dry mixture about ¼" thick. Sprinkle nuts over date filling, lightly pressing them into filling. Press remainder of dry mixture evenly on top.

Bake in 350°F. oven for 12-15 minutes. Chill and cut into squares for serving. Serve with mix of fresh or frozen peaches and rasberries.

Yield: 1 9 x 11 baking dish of date bars.

Banana-Date Cookies

3 bananas
1 cup chopped dates
⅓ cup oil
½ cup chopped walnuts
½ teaspoon salt
1 teaspoon vanilla
2 cups rolled oats

Mash bananas, leaving some pieces. Add chopped dates and oil. Beat with a fork. Add remaining ingredients. Mix lightly. Let stand for a few minutes for oatmeal to absorb moisture.

Drop from spoon on ungreased cookie sheet. Heat oven to 400°F. Bake 25 minutes or until nicely browned. Loosen with spatula and let cool on cookie sheet.

Yield: 24 cookies.

Whole Wheat Pie Crust

½ cup corn oil
½ cup water
1 teaspoon salt
2 cups whole wheat pastry flour (may substitute 1 cup quick oats if desired)

Beat oil and water with fork until creamy. Add salt and flour. Roll between waxed paper. Remove top piece of waxed paper and invert pie pan on crust. Quickly turn pan over with crust and waxed paper. Shape crust and paper into pan. Remove waxed paper. Bake at 425° for about ten minutes.

Apple Pie

6 cups apples, peeled and sliced
1 can (12 ounce) frozen apple juice, unsweetened
2 tablespoons cornstarch
1 teaspoon fennel seed (optional)
⅛ teaspoon salt

Simmer together until thickened. Pour into pie shell. Bake at 375°F. for 25 minutes or until done.

Carob Cream Pie

2 cups boiling water
½ cup raw cashews
20 large pitted dates
1 tablespoon vanilla
3 tablespoons carob powder
½ teaspoon salt
¼ cup cold water
¼ cup cornstarch
Whole Wheat Pie Crust, cooked and cooled
1-2 bananas
2 tablespoons flaked coconut

Mix boiling water and cashews in blender until smooth. Then add dates, vanilla, carob powder, and salt. Blend again. Pour into saucepan and bring to boil, stirring constantly to prevent scorching. Combine cold water and cornstarch in small bowl and mix well. Pour mixture into hot mixture, stirring vigorously to distribute quickly and evenly. As mixture begins to thicken, stir gently to prevent scorching. Cook about 1 minute until thick. Slice half the bananas lengthwise into cooled Whole Wheat Pie Crust. Pour filling into pie shell to cover bananas. Add another layer of bananas and cover with filling. Cool 15-20 minutes. Garnish with flaked coconut or scored banana, sliced diagonally and arranged in flower petal fashion in center of pie. Cool 1 hour at room temperature. Refrigerate at least 3 hours before serving. This could also be served without the pie shell as a custard or pudding in a parfait glass.

Raisin Tarts

Pastry Shells

¼ teaspoon salt
1 cup whole wheat pastry flour
1 teaspoon liquid lecithin
2 tablespoons water
¼ cup oil

Stir salt into flour. Mix liquid lecithin, water, oil with fork. Add liquid to the dry ingredients. If too dry, add a little more water. Press into muffin tin. Makes 7 tarts.

Filling

1 cup raisins
2 cups water
1 teaspoon cornstarch
2 teaspoons cold water
1 teaspoon vanilla

Boil raisins in water for 5-6 minutes. Make cornstarch solution and stir in with raisins after they've been cooked. Cook until thickens. Add vanilla after removed from the stove. Fill tart shells. Bake at 350°F. 15 minutes.

Variations:

1. Use a little lemon juice.
2. Cook with any unsweetened fruit juice rather than water
3. Add chopped nuts to top.

How to Cook Dry Beans and Peas

Amount Legume	Amount Water	Method	Amount Salt	Additional Seasoning (optional)	Amount Time	Amount Yield
1 cup beans	4 cups	Add to boiling water; as soon as beans boil again, turn off heat. Let stand 1 hour. Simmer until nearly done. Add salt. Continue cooking until beans are soft.	1 teaspoon	Sautéed onion in a little oil, a pinch of sweet basil, tomato puree, Baco Snacks, oregano, dill, savory, cumin	1–2 hours depending upon variety	2–2½ cups
1 cup soybeans or garbanzos	4 cups	Same as for beans. (Freezing after will shorten cooking time.)	1 teaspoon	As desired	2 hours or until tender	2–2½ cups
1 cup lentils or split peas	3 cups	Add to boiling water. Simmer until nearly done. Add salt and finish cooking.	3/4 teaspoon	As desired	15–30 minutes	2½ cups

References

Books by Ellen G. White include: *Counsels on Health, Counsels on Diet and Foods, Medical Ministry, Ministry of Healing, Testimonies;* Mountain View, California: Pacific Press Publishing Association; and Washington, D.C.: Review and Herald Publishing Association.)

(*How To Live* is a compilation of various articles on health, not generally available. Quotations from Ellen G. White listed here also appear in *Selected Messages,* available from the publishing houses shown above. **Help in Daily Living* is a reprint from *Ministry of Healing,* beginning at p. 469.)

Chapter 1

1. Testimonies, 2:64
2. Counsels on Health, p. 133
3. Counsels on Diet and Foods, p. 388

Chapter 2

1. Testimonies, 2:64
2. *Ibid.,* 2:368-69
3. Senate Select Committee Report, "Dietary Goals for the United States," p. 45.
4. *Ibid.,* p. 44
5. *Ibid.*
6. D. P. Burkett and H. C. Trowell, eds., *Refined Carbohydrate Foods and Disease.* London: Academic Press, 1975.
7. Senate Select Committee Report, "Dietary Goals for the United States," p. 33.
8. *Ibid.,* p. 13.
9. Inter-Society Commission Report, 1970.
10. Senate Select Committee Report, "Dietary Goals for the United States," p. 3.

11. Counsels on Health, p. 133
12. How To Live, p. 194★
13. Counsels on Diet and Foods, p. 388
14. *Ibid.,* p. 412
15. *Ibid.,* p. 385
16. *Ibid.,* p. 394
17. Help in Daily Living, p. 100★★
18. Testimonies, 2:68
19. Ministry of Healing, p. 302

Chapter 3

1. Counsels on Diet and Foods, p. 313
2. Senate Select Committee Report, "Dietary Goals for the United States," p. 17.
3. *Ibid.*
4. *Ibid.,* p. 4
5. Counsels on Diet and Foods, p. 312
6. Ministry of Healing, pp. 331-32
7. Counsels on Diet and Foods, p. 312
8. *Ibid.,* p. 349
9. *Ibid.,* p. 364
10. Counsels on Health, p. 117
11. Counsels on Diet and Foods, p. 313
12. *Ibid.,* p. 320
13. *Ibid.,* p. 321
14. *Ibid.*
15. *Ibid.,* p. 309
16. *Ibid.*
17. Testimonies, 1:681–82.
18. Counsels on Diet and Foods, p. 112
19. *Ibid.,* p. 411
20. *Ibid.,* p. 251
21. *Ibid.,* p. 260
22. *ibid.,* p. 258
23. *Ibid.,* pp. 258-59
24. *Ibid.,* p. 106
25. *Ibid.*
26. How To Live, p. 91★
27. Counsels on Diet and Foods, p. 85
28. Counsels on Health, p. 63

29. *Ibid.,* p. 147
30. Testimonies, 2:365
31. Ministry of Healing, p. 306
32. How To Live, p. 50★
33. Counsels on Diet and Foods, p. 105
34. Robert S. Goodhart and Maurice E. Shils, eds., "Modern Nutrition in Health and Disease: Dietotherapy." 5th ed. Philadelphia: Lea & Febiger, 1973, p. 948.
35. *Dental Survey,* April 1961, p. 475
36. *Journal of the American Dietetic Association,* 37:137-40, August, 1960.
37. Counsels on Diet and Foods, p. 138
38. *Ibid.,* p. 139

Chapter 4

1. How To Live, p. 171★
2. *Ibid.,* p. 177
3. *Ibid.*
4. *Ibid.,* p. 229
5. *Ibid.,* p. 212
6. *Loma Linda University Observer,* August 16, 1979
7. Testimonies, 3:490
8. How To Live, p. 127★
9. *Journal of Michigan State Medical Society.* 56:5, May, 1957, p. 599.
10. *Ibid.,* p. 591
11. *Ibid.,* p. 593
12. How To Live, p. 137★
13. *Ibid.*
14. *Ibid.,* pp. 137-38
15. *Ibid.,* p. 129
16. Counsels on Health, p. 193
17. *The Health Life,* Time–Life Special Report, 1966, p. 36.
18. Counsels on Health, p. 201; Testimonies, 4:94–95.
19. *Ibid.,* p. 104
20. *Ibid.*
21. How To Live, p. 124★
22. *Ibid.,* p. 186
23. *Ibid.,* p. 181
24. Counsels on Health, p. 84
25. Ministry of Healing, p. 327
26. *Cancer Facts and Figures,* American Cancer Society, 1978, p. 19.

27. Ministry of Healing, pp. 327–28
28. Counsels on Health, pp. 87–88
29. *Ibid.*, p. 441
30. *Medical World News,* March 19, 1979, pp. 11–12; quoted in *Echoes,* Fall, 1979.
31. Counsels on Diet and Foods, p. 442
32. Res. Rept. 2, AHA 5th Writers Forum, p. 15.
33. Medical Ministry, p. 11
34. Testimonies, 3:568
35. *Readers Digest,* December, 1979
36. Counsels on Health, p. 124
37. *Ibid.*, p. 174

Other Books

Published by Woodbridge Press Publishing Company
Post Office Box 6189, Santa Barbara, California 93111

(Please send amount shown plus 75¢ packing and shipping for first book; 40¢ each additional book ordered at the same time.)

The Oats, Peas, Beans & Barley Cookbook
By Edyth Young Cottrell, a complete vegetarian cookbook from a Loma Linda University research nutritionist. $4.95.

Stretching-the-Food-Dollar-Cookbook
By Edyth Young Cottrell. Vegetarian menus using nature's most economical foods. $3.95.

A Vegetarian Diet: How To Make It Healthful and Enjoyable
By Shirley T. Moore and Mary G. Byers, nutritionist and home economist. $3.95.

Problems With Meat
John A. Scharffenberg, M.D. Scientific analysis of dietary approaches using both meat and non-meat food products. $3.95.

Guide To Nutritional Factors in Foods
David A. Phillips. Analysis of foods with emphasis on natural products. $3.95.

How To Survive Snack Attacks—Naturally
By Judi and Shari Zucker. Healthful treats for both young and old. $3.95.

Books from Other Publishers

Nutrition for a Better Life
By Nan Bronfen, nutritionist for the Pritikin Research Foundation. $8.95. Capra Press, Santa Barbara, California 93101.

The Vegetarian Alternative
Sussman. $6.95. Rodale Press, Emmaus, Pennsylvania 18049.

It's Your World Vegetarian Cookery
Sponsored by Seventh-day Adventist Church. $3.50. Southern California Conference, Box 969, Glendale, California 91209.

375 Meatless Recipes: Century 21 Cookbook
By Ethel R. Nelson, M.D. $3.95. Eusey Press, 27 Nashau, Leamington, Massachusetts 01453.

Nature's Harvest
Walla Walla General Hospital Auxiliary. $5.95. College Place, Washington 99324.